Peppermint Bon Bons

Peppermint Bon Bons

Jacintha J. Canary

Copyright © 2011 by Jacintha J. Canary.

Library of Congress Control Number: 2011904344
ISBN: Hardcover   978-1-4568-8909-8
               Softcover   978-1-4568-8908-1
               Ebook   978-1-4568-8910-4

All rights reserved. No part of this book may be reproduced or transmitted in any form or by any means, electronic or mechanical, including photocopying, recording, or by any information storage and retrieval system, without permission in writing from the copyright owner.

This book was printed in the United States of America.

To order additional copies of this book, contact:
Xlibris Corporation
0-800-644-6988
www.xlibrispublishing.co.uk
Orders@xlibrispublishing.co.uk
301768

Contents

Acknowledgements 9

PART 1

Gadget Girl (Kuwait) (January 1990-present) 15
Ouma Betty (Ouma means Grandmother in Afrikaans) (1972-1986) 18
Potter Girl (November 2006) 21
Mum (1972-1999) 26
My Jamaican Homies (Summer 2006-present) 29
Oupa Ben (1980) 34
Beautiful Butterflies (2007-present) 36
Neighbourly Love (1981) 40
Dad (1972-2009) 43
Dad (May 2009-present) 46
Life or No Life (1972-1986) 48
Best Friend (1986-present) 53
College (January 1990-November 1993) 60
Past Relationships 62
Wedding Bells from Scotland (September 1996-December 1996) 70

PART 2

Life in the UK (February 1997) 77
A Break in Edinburgh, Scotland (April 1997) 80

Re-locating to Edinburgh (December 1997) 85
A Sudden Goodbye (November 1999) 89
Becoming a Mother (October 2000) 92
Depression (September 2003-present) 96
Restoration (September 2004-November 2010) 100
Gadget Girl 116
Sexual abuse 124

Afterword 127

This book is dedicated to my children Sophia and Lemoni

Acknowledgements

In starting this book it took me about 3months after my dad's death as I promised myself that when dad died I want no more secrets in my life.

Firstly I want to THANK GOD for bringing me to this point and using me to HEAL and draw strength from my past experiences.

My two beautiful daughters Sophia (my beautiful, creative reminder and sensitive, thoughtful spirit) and Lemoni (my burst of belief (little Lemon) and reminder of life as an adventure).

My sister (Carmelita Meyer), my brother-in-law (Felix Meyer), my nieces (Leigh, Caylan and Lindy Meyer for their joy, laughter and feisty spirits) my brothers (Nathaniel Canary and Malcolm Canary)

My Saheli sisters who have kept me strong and motivated with support of cakes, chocolate, laughter, tears and a connectedness during my time with Saheliya

Bertha Williams (My Engel) for cooking lovely lamb chops with onions and sugar (Cape Town style) and long chats at the weekends when we talked and talked about the lives we deserved.

Amy Westendarp for coffees intertwined with encouragement and gentle reminders to believe that I am amazing.

Adebanji (my companion) for being alongside me, for being patient with me.

Tersia Assumption my friend from College for all the long phone calls and encouraging talks late at night when I feel like this is really not worth it any more.

Janice Warmberg (South Africa), Leonie Sole (New Zealand), Gail and Ashwari for seeing positivity when I could not even bare to look at myself and think anything remotely positive.

Frank Daley and Theresa Clarke-Daley my friends that stood by me through thick and thin and lots of Wednesday and Sunday meals and Amadea my god daughter (my reminder to laugh, enjoy and laugh some more)

Buumba Mweetwa for messages of strength and support in moments of weakness.

Yvette Hunwick for her lessons in baking and support to keep me going to the gym to shift my relationship with myself and my body.

Carmen Kammies for always reminding me how great person I am and not some messed-up and abused victim gone off the rails. (Passed on in 1997)

Emily Dodd for your strength and unfailing Faith and belief in GOD and me even though I still struggle to accept acknowledgement for it. I am a work in progress like your butterfly.

Andrea Brown for our Tuesday talks and gifts of womanly wisdom in GOD . . . and of course the lovely cakes and soups (Yum Yum)

Wallace House staff at the time when I was suffering from Post-natal depression and met you amazing ladies who also did an amazing job in looking after my two beautiful children which I could not appreciate at the time because of the depression.

Canongate Youth Project (CYP), Multicultural Family Base (MCFB),SAHELIYA, Link-Up Women's Support Centre, Women Onto Work (WOW),Women Supporting Women (Pilton Health Project) and SHAKTI Women's Aid.

Caryn Abrahams for getting me into grounded and focus-mode and keeping me on the track even though many times I felt like it was too difficult and not interested to stay on the PATH with GOD.

Takako for her wit sensitivity and inspirational talks when things seem really TOO MUCH at the time.

My home group for the support and nurturing you have given me all the time and your patience with all my questions and stories about life. DESTINY CHURCH and it's members (staff and non-staff) for your openness and acceptance to all of us who have strayed onto The path and stuck with us through the UPS AND DOWNS of becoming a stronger Christian.

A thank you to all of you who have come onto my path, touched my life and have contributed to my recovery.

PART 1

Gadget Girl (Kuwait) (January 1990-present)

. . . .

Present

(Telephone conversation between Jacintha and Tersia) The friends speak about once a month on average, but also texts over the weeks as well as Facebook.)

J—What are you up to?

T—"I m getting my I-phone sorted it is driving me mad, but I still love it!!"

J—You know what I think right. (I'll say it anyway) I think it is overly expensive and way too complicated, who wants to receive and send emails from their mobile?

T—yeah yeah mother dear . . . .

J—you love your comforts, fast car, fancy clothes, expensive perfume and your appreciation of the opposite species. That's why we are friends. You are the woman I wish to be and I am the sensible woman you wish you were . . . sometimes . . . oh alrite never.

T—F . . . k th_t, but something along those lines.

J—You know I like you right and the fact that my mum never liked you made me even more determined to be your friend right?

T—Something like that yeah. Your sister still thinks that we are always up to no good.

J—I know that is why it is so funny because people always think the worst of us.

T—I am so overweight!!! This stomach must go it is getting on my nerves.

But the dude says it is nice and he likes it, makes me look like a woman and not the skinny girl I used to be.

J—I agree with the dude, a little bit of excess curves are great. Too skinny would not work . . . .

T—Do you remember the good old college days? When you used to skip classes and never turn up?

J—Yes and I failed my first year because of my bad attitude and you never got your bursary until the final year because your attendance was dodgy?

T—How are the kids doing?

J—They are good, your" child "(Lemoni) is up to her usual, full of life and has an answer for everything and Sophia is here very much getting into cooking and wanting to make cups of tea. She is lovely really, but your child is taking advantage of her kind nature and I have to step in or else she will get Sophia to do everything for her . . . .

T—How is the book coming on?

J—Been tough looking at the old stuff, but it is getting there. I want to launch it this year November (2010) but if not It will have to coincide with April next year (2011).

T—Okay that's good and you know where I am if you need to talk, but I have to dash, give my children a hug each!! (Ek het nie f____n lus vir die skool nie, mense maak my siek) Bye . . . bye . . . enjoy jou dag more!!

J—okay thanks for the call and thanks for your 110 percent friendship . . . bye . . . bye

Ouma Betty (Ouma means Grandmother in Afrikaans) (1972-1986)

....

My grandmother taught me how to embroider and sew drawstring bags with the leftover fabric and clothes people left on the buses where my grandfather cleaned the buses. Whatever people left on the buses and did not claim in a month's time, grandfather would bring to my grandmother. She would then teach me how to make beautiful little drawstring bags in the most amazing colours and fabrics.

You see, that was my special time as my mum and I never really had a connection, so I loved spending time with my OUMA (Grandmother). At the age of 9 onwards I started wetting the bed, the doctor put it down as me being an anxious child. I would dream that I would be going to the toilet and then wake up soaking wet and smelling of pee (urine). Mum did not like this at all and tried all sorts of ways to make me stop drinking any drinks at 6:30pm, she would wake me up when they went to bed, but I still wet the bed. When I went to Ouma Betty's, I tried not to wet the bed. I went to do the potty (as in those days the bathroom and toilet was outside and a long way away from the main house. Ouma Betty too would wake me in the middle of the night to make me go and pee, but I still wet the bed. Even when I did wet the bed, Ouma Betty was a wee bit upset, but not quite volcanic as mum. Mum would start shouting at me: "take of the covers, take the wet mattress outside and put it in the front so everyone can see that you wet the bed, as it was a nuisance and I should be old enough to go to the toilet in the night."

I continued wetting the bed way into my teens up to 18 I guess. My Ouma Betty accepted me for who I was and did not try to change me. I love her for that and this love has pulled me through the pits of depression, sadness, hurt, loss, guilt, anger and indecision.

I always remember her loving brown eyes, lovely smooth light brown skin, soft and silky black hair with lots of grey in it pleated neatly and lying over her shoulder. She used to get me to brush it and plait it and also to pull out the grey hairs.

She was a Tamal Indian who married a coloured boy which was unheard of, left her family and set out to start her own family. She had 10 children, 4 boys and 6 girls (lost one baby). She became a Catholic late in life I must have been 11 or 12. She always told me to pray; "Jesus, Mary and Joseph please help me," if I ever felt scared or needed help in school with my exams or in the night time.

This little prayer helped me through a lot of close-calls in life.

You see, I believe GOD puts people in your path when you need them and when you are ready for a new connection.

Ouma Betty smelt like "Amla" oil and peppermint. When I went round to visit and sleepover, we would get up early, get washed, soak the washing in the big bath tubs, soak it with "Omo" washing powder (and later on I would go stamp up and down with my cousin Hayley until our feet were all wrinkly and soft) then go into the kitchen where she would make the "mieliemeel/mealie-meal pap"(maize meal). I can still smell the mieliemeel cooking as if I am there in the house at number 10 Curtis Street, Korsten, Port Elizabeth, she would make it thick and lumpy, just the way I like it. She would then add "Rama" margarine, "Hulletts" white sugar and "Steri milk"(full fat of course). Yum yum . . . I would scoff it down under her watchful eyes. She had two quarter pieces of white fresh "Britos" bread with a thin scraping of Rama and a cup of weak Rooibos tea with a half a teaspoonful of sugar every morning and every evening before she went to bed (sometimes I would make the bread and tea for her when I stayed over).

She had a mean side to her too when she would be shouting at the children(my siblings and cousins), but luckily for me I did not get to see that side of her very often. In the late morning we would go and make the beds and after that usually she would get me to brush her hair and pull out the grey ones. Sometimes I told her that there were not any more left as there were loads and I was looking forward to my peppermint bon bon which she kept wrapped up in her special handkerchief in her wardrobe.

I would like to think that these peppermint bon bons were only for the special ones-
(grandkids who earned it or who had a special place in Ouma Betty's life).

Potter Girl (November 2006)

....

(Yvette and Jacintha having a meal at Jacintha's house)

Entrance: Y coming in looking very beautiful with her hair pulled back and her big, beautiful eyes are shining, her skin is radiant and she is wearing a cool black sweater and a faded and washed out, trendy jeans with a hole above the right knee. Her body is immaculate because of all the work outs at the gym and her very disciplined attitude to healthy eating.

J—Hey how are you doing? Looking Good as always!! How is the dude???

Y—You know I just do not feel it, but thanks my friend. Oh my man is seriously bad. I will tell you later. How are you and how is your man??

J—I am getting excited as we have been chatting for a while now and I think I am beginning to understand a little bit about him . . . as much as I can with what cross-Atlantic communication allows. I like him, I just have to meet him now . . . . I think I asked God for a soul mate and he near enough almost someone similar to me which is quite scary, but also reassuring . . . . Does that make sense?? You know how I am around men . . .

Y—Yes you mean your huge hang-ups around trust issues????? You know.

J—Yes I know and I feel sometimes I am ready and sometimes I just do not want to get out there, yet this year I am taking more risks. Sensible risks I might add.

Y—Jazzy you are beautiful and such a kind spirit, I wish you would find a lovely dude as you so deserve a nice guy.

J—I would love one and this year I feel different so I wish God would send me someone kind, loving, supportive and smart mostly, but He must love God and also be willing to support me in the work I have to do with women and men.

Y—Jazzy, I sure hope that you meet him, I have to vet him first of course I do not want you to get hurt. (moves into the kitchen and sorts out fish to be defrosted) This smells yummy.

J—Would you like a hot drink? Rooibos*, Berry or Peppermint?

Oh I love the heart bowl You made me for Christmas, I have been using it for everything, my cereal, my dessert, snacks and more . . . . The girls know that it is my special bowl and not to touch it . . .

Y—Rooibos please? I am glad you love it!

J—(makes tea while Yvette defrosts the fish in the microwave.) What will I do with this fish as I normally just do a foil job, spice for fish, herbs, close the foil and put it in the oven for 20 to 30 minutes.

Y—(takes her tea) I usually pour oil on, spice it, lots of salt and bake for 30 minutes, then grill for 5 to 10 minutes. (let's go through to the living room and catch up)

J—Okay I will do that, let's go through to the living room.

(both ladies go through to the living room and have a seat on the sofas across from each other)

J—Would you like some wine? I feel for some, but I do not want to drink it all as I only like a little bit, would you like to take the rest with you?

---

* South African caffeine-free tea with anti-oxidants and minerals

Y—I would love some! A small amount for me as well please.

(Jacintha goes through to the kitchen to get the wine and two glasses from the cupboard and returns with it)

J—So tell me about the dude, you look tired.

Y—He came down the other day and we talked.

J—What, that is what you wanted all along?

Y—That is exactly what I said to him, but he could not see it.

J—And how are you feeling now?

Y—Girl I am shattered and I still feel numb. Can you check the fish I am starving?

J—goes through to the kitchen and checks fish, comes through and shows Yvette.

Y—Put it under the grill now then we could have it in ten minutes or so.

J—(Goes back through to the kitchen and puts fish back under the grill) It looks good I would never grill it, but Now I can try something different with my fish next time. Where were we?

Y—The dude . . . . I just do not know, I invested so much time in this man and I still hope that he can come round and find something in him of what he showed to be.

J—Yes and I hope that he can see that because he actually did not even give anything to you, it was all on his terms . . .

Y—Thank you my friend, now tell me about your dude you have been chatting to?

J—Later let's get the food on and enjoy the wine.

(they go through to the kitchen and bring through the beetroot, avocado and lettuce salad, spiced and grilled sea bass fish, basmati rice and stir fried vegetables)

Washed down with A lovely South African red wine.

J—Yeah, do not know, we have been chatting since 2nd of January so it has been a month now, I get a good sense of him, but also I think he has been hurt a lot in the past and he . . . , he is fussy, likes to go and spend time by himself, does not want to be smothered . . . do you see the similarities. It was like I am telling my own profile.

Y—You know! You are so funny you just pretend that you do not like it, but deep down you probably would be just fine because you are so alike.

J—I would hate to disagree but I actually agree. I feel excited, but I also know I HAVE TO BE CAUTIOUS.

Y—I have to come and check him out when you meet him . . .

J—Yes, you and Frank.

Y—Sure my friend, now that was yummy.

J—Thank you, dessert is watermelon and melon.

Y—Thanks but I am stuffed just now. Let's go and get a hot drink and watch the movie.

J—Okay, Berry or Peppermint?

Y—Berry please.

J—Okay. (clears the dishes away with Yvette and gets the tea made) I will finish up here, you go and make yourself comfortable and I will come through.

(They chat some more then watches the movie—"Diary Of A Mad Black Woman while munching on some dried fruit and nuts)

Later like 10:30pm Yvette offers to do the dishes, but Jacintha stops her.

J—You have to go as I have to talk to the dude, I have to be honest as I AM REALLY LOOKING FORWARD TO TALKING TO HIM AS I AM AWAY TILL SUNDAY FOR MY COUNSELLING RESIDENTIAL WEEKEND!!!

Please Go!!

Y—Okay thanks for your honesty, I get your message and I appreciate it that you can tell me to go. (hugs Jazz and goes out the front door with a cheeky grin on her face)

Mum (1972-1999)

What I remember about my mum is that she never hugged me, told me that I was beautiful or gave me any compliments like: "You look pretty today"; "That dress sits lovely on you"; "Well done Jacintha". Mum took me to school on the first day of school at the age of 4 and a half and the next day I walked to school with my brother.

The bedwetting experiences was beginning to get more frequent from my 9th birthday onwards. Mum continued shouting at me in the mornings."Why didn't you get up when you felt the pee coming?" Truth is I never felt it, I dreamt I was in the bathroom doing my business, I would feel the warm sensation and then be too scared to get up to go to the toilet to get cleaned up. Mum made me take of the sheets, soak them in the big plastic buckets and then I had to put the wet stinking mattress outside by the front wall where all the kids from the neighbourhood could see me put it out. "I was so shy, this made me cringe with embarrassment and shame, sometimes I tried to put it at the back if Mum was not around or if she was on a nightshift meaning she would only go straight to bed and wake up much later in the day. Sometimes she would make me shift it back to the front, in the middle of the day in sight of all the young boys. The boys would tease me, call me names that I could find too embarrassing to mention here.

Mum never went to one of our parent evenings and never came to watch us play sports, I guess looking back now she was too busy working hard to make ends meet and clothe four children and a sick husband.

She never showed any emotions in line with love, warmth and kindness, it was always straight-faced, stern and a no-nonsense expression. My friends were all scared of her. Nobody messed with Sophy Canary and all the kids in the street stayed well away from Mrs. Canary's. No children came round to play as we were kept in our yard and only played with each other. We hardly ever went to the park, when we did, we had to leave early in order to get home before mum knew we were at the Park. I remember the swings vividly; I would feel free and forget about everything when I was on the swings, I felt like I was dreaming of floating back and forth, back and forth . . . .

So much so that I woke up on the ground. This happened a couple of times; I would fall on my face. Looking back I felt I was escaping all the feelings I was struggling with: I was too shy, too nervous, too quiet, too clumsy, too gentle, too soft according to My Mother which were all signs of weakness. We were taken to Church every Sunday, dressed in our best clothes, have lovely food and then would go to "Ouma Betty's". That was the best part of the day, because I could hang out with my cousin Hayley who was 1 and a half years younger than me. Haley was the daughter of my Uncle (Mum's eldest brother). Her mum was not my mum's favourite person. I was told to stay away from Hayley, but I loved going there, there was no pressure and we could eat what we wanted any time, this was great!!!! My aunt loved me and treated me like one of her own, she always hugged me when she saw me. Hayley's mum also made our hair pretty at Christmas times—it would get chemically straightened with straightening cream, neutralised, washed, conditioned, set in rollers and be absolutely beautiful and soft the next day and for a month thereafter. I even got to sleep at Ouma Betty's on these nights which meant I was away from mum and had more time with my cousin Hayley, more playtime and girly time. I could hardly contain myself.

Christmases would be spent at Ouma Betty's where there would be food, food and more food . . . : ox tongue, salted Beef, Leg of lamb, Gammon, curry, beetroot salad (sweet and sour), baked beans salad, potato salad, carrot and pine apple salad, cucumber salad, trifle, fridge tart, fruit cake, sponge cake, peppermint tart and much much more in the way of savoury snacks: samoosas, mince pies and more . . . . Yum Yum, those were happy days.

My Jamaican Homies (Summer 2006-present)

. . . .

(I have known them for over 4 years now, yet it feels like a lifetime. They have listened to my stories patiently and I have listened to theirs on many occasions usually involving very tasty cooked food and sometimes washed down with a good bottle of wine. My Jamaican Homies, Frank, Theresa and Amadea (My goddaughter)

We regularly meet up for fellowship and often eat together as food seem to be pivotal to our sharing and we have a lot of good family memories surrounding food and togetherness.)

Frank—Jacintha it is good to see you, how are you?(big hug)

Jacintha—Good to see you too Frank, what's up?

F—things are good

J—Hi Theresa (big hug)

Theresa—Hi Jay, you look beautiful.

J—Thank you Theresa, how has your week been, how's work?

Amadea—Hi Aunty Jay! (big voice and a lovely smile)

J—Hi Amadea (big hug and a kiss on the cheek) It's good to see you Amadea, what would you like to drink Tootsie?

(the adults go through to the livingroom and chat, the girls either play outside or in their room and come through for snacks and drinks)

I met Theresa at a Summer event for volunteers. I liked her easiness and relaxing demeanour. Her little girl Amadea was about 2 and a bit and she told me that they recently moved from Skye (Up North). My first thoughts were, oh my goodness she has been exposed to poor treatment up there because there is not many black people up that part of the world. We exchanged mobile numbers and left it at that. That same night I bumped into a lady that attended the same organisation around the same time when I was receiving Complimentary Therapies and Counselling for a period while I was looking at my relationship with my ex-husband at the time. I had Sophia (four at the time) and Lemoni two and a half). This lady at the time was really someone I admired as her makeup was always flawless and she looked like someone I could never be friends with and I never thought of approaching her then. It turned out that she thought the same of me at the time . . .

That night she invited me to stay behind for a service after the event, I did not want to stay as I did not feel close to God at all and I guess I was angry that I had to be alone and that God was nowhere in sight. She kept my handbag to ensure that I stayed, needless to say I felt uncomfortable, firstly because I was being forced and did not have a choice and secondly it was very free and she kept my handbag so I was left powerless and frustrated.

Theresa and I never saw each other again, but we bumped into each other on a bus in August sometime while I was taking Lemoni to the Roundabout group where she went to a multicultural crèche for under fives. I also met Frank that day (I guess we were sort of checking each other out to see if we were for real). Frank and I were similar in many ways, we assess within the first few minutes and check whether this person evokes good or bad vibes and then go with what our gut senses.

We ended up living ten minutes from each other and started introducing Wednesday night meals and Sunday lunches and just when we wanted to hang out really. Theresa is about 5 foot 5, with beautiful brown skin and lovely dark brown eyes, her make-up is always applied well, has a lovely well shaped body and dresses really trendy. She always tells me that I look nice and that I am beautiful. I never felt I deserved these compliments because my image of myself is so low, but I never said that out loud, I guess the uncomfortable way I accept these compliments tell their own story. It wasn't until recently that I had Theresa over for a meal one night and I told her that I really appreciate her compliments, but I could never accept it because I do not see myself as beautiful, because my parents never gave us compliments. In her usual lovely, warm manner Theresa has taught me to accept my beauty and that it does not mean that I am unlovable or ugly at all and that I am worthy of receiving compliments.

Theresa and I went to The Shakti 21st year celebration together, the first evening gown I had worn since I left my marriage, and I felt and looked great! Yvette was also there, along with a fellow South African friend and a lot of other prominent women who has made my journey worthwhile.

Our children are growing up together and they are learning about closeness and kinship in their own way. They are after all family through our connections.

The girls played well together and we had our first New Year's meal at The Hard Rock Cafe (1st January 2007) in George Street and celebrated Amadea's, Theresa's and Lemoni's birthday. It was lovely to spend time together.

A few years later Theresa and Frank asked me to be Amadea's godmother and my first thought was (s__t, I am not a Christian and oh dear I will have to be responsible to this little person and I have to look at my own relationship with God).But Frank and Theresa took it in their stride and worked with me on my insecurities around my Faith and hung in there with me. Theresa is so lovely and so accepting of me I had a few hang-ups around her relaxed attitude with time, but we have now worked on it so I guess I have learnt a few things from her. She has a lovely manner with the children and she is great with fashion and style, she has kept me on my toes and always has a good few compliments to give even though I did not always receive it well. Theresa also asked me to be her bridesmaid a year and a half ago and I was really honoured to be asked to be this close to someone I have become to really get close to. I had seen her truly stand rock-solid in her walk with God and how she truly lives being unconditional with everyone. She is always ready to help out and to listen when I felt really helpless . . . .

When I think of Frank I think of him as a gentle, dependable, consistent, well dressed and stylish friend who is like a brother to me and someone I think of as reliable.

Frank has had his own struggles, but he never shows any of this and is a true gentleman. Frank is about 5 foot 7, brown-skinned, gentle dark brown eyes, broad shoulders and a smile that lights up his face, yet very humble and self-controlled. I say self-controlled because he never gives any emotions away. I guess I say that because it is such a big thing for me to trust men in general and my connections and attitudes about men has been tainted and scarred because of my earlier connections with the men in my life as a girl and young woman. In many ways he reminds me of my grandfather who got the job done and made no big fuss about it. He is calm, quiet, yet confident even if it looks like he is not taking any notice at all. Sophia, my eldest daughter is close to him as I think they share a similar spirit. Quietly observing and feeling things first before jumping in as I would say. Frank took a while before he warmed up to me and vice versa as we are too very much similar in many ways. Your word is your bond; and you do not ask unnecessarily; and you plan things in advance are kind of the stuff of Frank's make-up. I will never forget this conversation shortly before my Baptism;(we were walking to the bus stop, Frank being the gentleman that he is had to walk me to the bus stop, see me get on the bus and then walk off), talking about the girls and life in general. He said to me:" I like the new you and I can see the changes in you for the better and I thank God for the change in you. He knew I had hang-ups and that also meant our friendship was at a whole new level of trust as I do not take feedback from just anyone or I will cut you down to size. Frank also dreamt about me making a decision to follow God and I thought oh well, that's great, but little did I know that God had other plans in store for me. Frank's objectivity and sense of calm has helped me from going off the rails and reacting and stopping me to think through things first before I go in all excited and reactive, but to think and then respond first instead of jumping in. Frank has been and still is a steady, calm, constant and supportive presence in my life.

Oupa Ben (1980)

Oupa Ben was a tall, dark-skinned and very upright man. I remember my grandfather's face was always looked permanently serious, although he had a gentle side to him too. He worked in a bus depot cleaning the buses. He would leave 4:00am in the morning and return to around 2:00pm in the afternoons. His back was always sore and ouma Betty or later one of the grandchildren had to rub it with Zambuck Ointment. It must have been all that bending over seats and washing those big double decker buses.

The good thing for us cousins were that Oupa Ben got free cinema passes for Saturdays and the holidays!! We had go in shifts as there were so many of us—one week the oldest girls and boys, next week the middle ones and the following week older cousins and little ones.

The little ones did not get to go much as they would not sit still for long and ended up fighting and falling asleep or wanting to go to the toilet all the time. It was mostly Charles Bronson movies, but I did not mind as the free pass also came with free sweets, juice and ice-cream and if you were smart you would make the big bag of sweets last two weeks.

Oupa Ben played on the horses and I remember him asking me to choose numbers for him, if he won I would get some money for myself. He also collected glass bottles, actually bought them—children would bring the bottles to him and he would pay them for it, then he would wash them, clean them and go and sell them at this huge, big place that had lots of bottles.

He always went once a month on those trips to the big warehouse place that he took the bottles to and sometimes one of the grandchildren would be allowed to go with him. Most of the time he took my oldest cousin with, because he was Oupa Ben's favourite, he knew about cars and most things Oupa Ben likes. On this one day, I got to go with. He drove a Cream Toyota Corolla "Bakkie", open back van without a canopy.

Oupa Ben loaded the "Bakkie" with the crates of bottles; there were green ones, brown ones, clear ones, blue ones and all sorts. I got to sit beside him in the front when we set off for Checkers Hypermarket. We walked in and I must have got lost along the way, all I knew is that I found myself wandering up and down in the car park trying to locate Oupa Ben's Bakkie. I was not crying or feeling any panic, but I could vaguely remember hearing my name over the microphone but did not hink anything of it, but I kept wandering around the car park, I found my way back in to the Customer Service desk where I found Oupa Ben with a lovely lady, who asked me if I was okay, where was I? My grandfather did not look pleased, but did not say anything either. We went home to Ouma Betty's, when we got there he relayed the story to everybody there and they all laughed at me. My cousins, the aunts and uncles, and my brothers and sister. The cousins teased me for a long time after that and Oupa Ben never took me anywhere with him again.

Beautiful Butterflies (2007-present)

. . . .

I started attending Destiny Church on an invitation from a former work colleague, Amy Watts (now Amy Westendarp) in February 2007. Amy and I used to have lots of chats at work about women's issues and we have hearts and passion for women I guess. I can remember lots of days we would chat about communities and how we are dissatisfied with how some communities get far less than others. I felt a connection with Amy and we also started meeting for coffees as coffee is always welcome; firstly to get out of the office and secondly just girly chats are great opportunities to chat and just be with your girl friend.I went on and off until April 2007 as I was still in two minds as to what I wanted to change about my life. I asked her some silly questions like: Will I get into trouble if I do not attend one Sunday and what if My kids are sick? Will they give me homework?;Will I get into trouble if I do not take my bible? Will they judge me or give me a hard time because I am divorced? All sorts of defensive questions I guess, looking back now.

Like they say, hindsight is a good thing!!!! (they were right, whoever they are)

They do this thing at the end where Pete (the Pastor at Destiny Church Edinburgh, who wears Converse trainers, jeans and a t-shirt) says a prayer for you to give your life to God in order to start afresh and accept God into your life (The Salvation Prayer). I did this a couple of times, the first few times I was very emotional and in a bad place emotionally, I guess. But after the fourth time I felt a difference in myself I guess and some of the guilt shifted. (I took God seriously I guess). A prayer person comes to pray with you and walks alongside you on your journey. That Sunday I was blessed and lucky to get a football-playing, blue-eyed, young looking girl called Emily. We went for a hot chocolate in a pub (I know, I thought all Christians were uptight, boring I told you so's and very un-fun) She was off to football afterwards and she did not even give me HOMEWORK!!! I thought this was a one-off, but hey I will be able to duck the next few meetings . . . We failed to get another suitable time to meet and then I bumped into her at my local Tesco's and she told me, she is moving into my neighbourhood and I told her : "Oh that's near me," without mentioning that it is actually five minutes from my house (Like I said, God really had other plans for me). Emily came over to my house on a regular basis, she met the girls and we have movie nights together and we share lots of times together. When the girls are at their dad's we hang out together, cook meals together, drink tea together, share happy times, stressful times, sad times, tearful times, and lots of positive times together.

I grew a lot in my Faith with Emily and our regular meetings, chats and sharing lots of good food.

I told Emily my sad story and she did not flinch at all or passed judgement, this really amazed me and Emily really showed that she is a true Christian (Initially I thought what can this 27 year old teach me? but boy did I learn a lit within the next two years about my walk with God and trusting in his plan. Emily's total commitment and her living out her faith daily has spurred me on to become even closer to God in order to have that hunger for God. She gives totally with the trust that God will provide for her every need. A lesson I had to learn from being in close proximity with Emily. At the time it wasn't always as straightforward as I said to Emily one evening, "bring it on God, I am ready". I then went through a period of disbelief and doubt I guess, I planned to get Baptised, but I kept ducking out of it. So Emily had to ask me straight up; What is going on tell me when you gonna do it, because I need to put it in my diary!!!"Bring it on . . . came to mind" yes God has a way of reminding you about things as you go along just as he promised, He does not like to be messed around with."

I got Baptised on Sunday the 13th of September 2009, a day that also made my walk with God quite visible to the Church community and my burial of my Past (although that last part proved to be much harder than I thought).

I joined the classes that enabled me to become a member of Destiny Ministries and served on the Team as a Trainee Counsellor at the church since April 2009 till present. Emily told me to speak to Roddy and offer my services and I probably still would not have done anything about it, if it wasn't for Emily's faith in my abilities as a person. Like Theresa, Emily saw something I did not accept in myself that I am worthy and quite capable.

She listened to me all the time when I was having a tough time at work and also as I was getting closer to God and also looking at my relationship with myself and my body and how she then used her all—accepting love to be with me through thick and thin (at the gym urging me on and motivating me to keep going when I feel like life is getting too much or I am doubting my abilities as a parent).

When I told Emily that I am writing my book she did not laugh at me and say: "what a stupid idea", instead she encouraged me to get started and she believed that my story will help lots of other women to come to receive Christ's Freedom as He did for me.

Emily is always talking about butterflies and their processes and I have come to associate her with beautiful, strong, yet sensitive butterflies who always hold their sensitivity well, whilst being strong enough to go out there and do their thing!!

She does not play football much now, we go to the gym and we go for lovely picnics and walks and we talk about all sorts of stuff and God of course. She surfs and goes snowboarding, cool indeed. Emily and I still meet up for coffees, lunches, basketball in the spring and summer, movie nights with the girls and walks.

'Awesome', 'Amazing' and 'Go for it': are some of her popular sayings and she totally is all that and more . . .

Neighbourly Love (1981)

. . . .

My brothers and I often played outside in the back garden because we were not allowed in the street or park with the other children. Malcolm, my youngest brother and I used to play well together. He had this little plastic dog with big Black Eyes and a ripple effect textured hair and fur which was painted, THAT HE TOOK EVERYWHERE HE WENT.

We also had new neighbours we could get to visit, so sometimes we would sneak out and go to see some of the neighbours that mum approved of. Some of them had all interesting things in their back gardens and sometimes we would be allowed to get some of the fruit and vegetables growing in the gardens like berries, carrots, figs and guavas. I can remember my brother and I going to this neighbour's house and we would play there mostly, we would get lots of sweets, biscuits and nice stuff. Then I also remembered my brother wander off and I would be left alone with this man who would always ask me, "what is the nicest thing?". I would answer "sweets ". Then he would say that he will show me what the nicest thing is. He would then take me to the bedroom and made to touch his penis, I would pull my hand away, but he would pull it and make me touch it and stroke it and sometimes put Vaseline on to make it slide easier. I remember wanting to pull away and get out of the room, but he would block me off and pull me back. Sometimes the games would involve him touching my vagina and even penetrating my privates (vagina). I would often be sick after these visits and would not have appetite for my dinner, but Mum would force me to finish my food. Each time I would try to get my brother to stay behind with me, but my loving neighbour had other plans in mind. He would be very good at giving my brother enough snacks and other stuff to keep him distracted and then my brother would disappear. I was told, "this is our secret, you will get in trouble if you tell anybody." I stopped going along after a long while, I must have been nine and a half at the time. I started wetting the bed all the time and have nightmares and strange dreams about running away and being chased by men in black coats and big black hats and I was scared that they would get me if I went to toilet in the middle of the night. I saw this man with a Black Top hat, Black Cape and Black trousers sitting at the end of my bed, he was watching me and because I had been a Naughty little girl. Mum shouted at me more and more, I wet the bed more and more and became quiet and more withdrawn. I started wetting myself in school because I was too scared to go and ask to go to toilet and was scared that the teacher would know that I am a naughty little girl. I would be so busy trying to pinch my legs together that I lost the sensation that told me when I needed to go to the toilet straight away. I started waking up in the middle of the night and wanting to go into my parents' bed. Mum said no, because I would get them wet and also my youngest brother's place, there was no space for me. Dad tried to speak to me, but by then I did not really trust either of them, let alone any adult I do not know. Nobody protected me and I thought I had to protect myself. There was also the constant little voice in the back of my head saying "they are going to beat you when they find out and you will get the blame because they will not believe that your neighbour was doing all this to you and why did you not come and tell us and why did you wait so long to tell us?"

I even started wetting myself in Church during the service, much to my mum's frustration. I remember this Saturday evening, we went to evening service. I was wearing a purple trousers and a black and white polo neck jumper. I wet myself during the service and even though I knew I had to go, I did not. Mum was furious and told me off and pinched my arm in the soft bit under the arm. This was my favourite trousers and I was scared that I would be going to Ouma Betty's after church and I would be smelling of Pee . . . .

Ouma Betty did not make a big deal and she gave me a towel to sit on and I think my cousin Hayley gave me a jeans to borrow. My brothers and sister chose to sit as far away from me as possible and teased me the whole time. I did not tell anyone about the secret touching sessions as I felt ashamed, no good, ugly and I felt Alone and dirty. I used to dream about flying over the desert and feeling free, but then I would wake up and realise it was just a dream and realise that the mattress is soaked with pee. I stopped going round to all the neighbours' houses and played in our own yard and mostly inside with my dolls. You see my body was changing, breasts were developing and my hips got round and all kinds of other stuff that I did not have control off.

I started stealing money from mum's wallet, silver coins at first then notes. I was buying sweets, crisps and treats for children in order to be my friends and for them to like me. I was doing exactly what my abuser taught me but just not the touching stuff. He gave me sweets; **Quality Streets** and **Roses" chocolates;** I cannot stand them till today as well as **Lemon Twist cooldrink.** Later on it was money, coins mostly never notes.

I thought that if you give people what they like, you will have plenty of friends.

Dad (1972-2009)

Dad was of White descent (White looking coloured), beautiful Italian features, dark eyes, Olive skin, pitch black wavy hair, a killer smile and a razor sharp brain.

One can see how mum fell for him. She always said that I look like him and I think my curly hair is courtesy of dad's gene line.

Dad was very strict, he trained as a teacher at teacher's college as it was what most of the family regarded as a respectable profession. I am never quite sure if he liked it or not, I never heard him say that.

I remember mum saying that dad was involved in a motorbike accident and it resulted in him not being able to do strenuous work as his spine was held together by a steel rod and metal pins. I cannot recall this event or if it was before or after they got married. Dad taught at some schools and covered as a temporary teacher for short periods, but never held any jobs down for long enough to be a steady source of income to compliment Mum's nurse's wage.

That meant that dad stayed at home and looked after us all mostly when he was not in-between jobs. We had a lot of jobs to do after we got in from school; polish our shoes, hang up of fold our school clothes, change into our normal clothes and then do our homework. Reading, Maths and Spelling were the most important ones. We had to write 10 new words from the dictionary, learn their meanings and copy them down and learn how to spell them as dad tested us on it as well. We had to learn our times tables and number bonds and then do our Maths homework. No praise was given or any signs of encouragement. "There's no such word as I can't do It", "Do it again"—still rings in my ears as a blast from the past. These messages still ring in my ears from time to time when I have to do anything remotely to do with anything academic, form filling or official letters and contracts. Dad did not talk much he had a way of saying something very slowly and loaded with . . . unsaid words or actions. I just knew that there will be serious consequences if I do not do what he asked us to.

This would be a physical punishment or criticism which still affects me at certain times in my life. Dad never used to hug me or sit me on his lap, the closest I got was family photos with all of us in our pyjamas, if I was lucky I would sit on his lap next to my youngest brother.

When I was 10 I started getting my hair chemically straightened with "Sheen", "Soft & Silky", "Wella" straightening Cream. This made my front dry afro hair very shiny and manageable.

At the time there was this advert for VO5. It was an advert for VO5 shampoo and conditioner making your hair soft, shiny and silky.

"Wow look at me now" Was the catchphrase. I remember this Saturday when I came home from "Pauline's" the hairdressers and the first thing my dad said was "wow look at me now". Now I did not know to take that as a compliment in stead I took it as embarrassment and a joke. I put my head down and ran to the room.

The repeating of the VO5 advert catchphrase was as close as I was ever going to get to a compliment from my dad. Around that time, I remember I started stealing food like apples, biscuits and half ate them in the middle of the night and then leave the rest tucked in among my clothes in the drawer. I also started stealing chewing gums, chocolates and small packets of sweets in supermarkets when we did the grocery shopping. I could sneak them in under my arms and in my trousers and in my panty. Mum noticed this and started to check my clothes after we went shopping and if she did find anything, I would get a beating from my dad. I was hoping to get caught as the memories of the abuse was eating away at me. I started cutting my hair as well as a punishment for the pain of the abuse and I knew if my hair was ugly and disgusting that would also make it true that I controlled that part of my body. I would also pull my hair out in clumps if and when someone paid me a compliment.

Dad taught my cousin and I at the age of three to plait and braid my little dolls hair. This was a soft side to him and at times I wished that he would show me that soft side especially when I was yearning and wasting away with sadness, guilt and shame on the inside. I was just a little girl wanting to be loved and protected and I cried at the bottom of their bed and sometimes I would almost say: "He did shameful and bad things to me and I can't sleep as I do not want to think about it any more, but I did not, in stead I cried softer and softer so no one can hear me. Inside I was screaming "I am scared, please, please help me. (I feel sad writing this, but I am not bursting into tears like I used to).When we did not listen or we were being naughty, dad used to beat us with a belt, an electric cord/cable and sometimes his bare hands which were very big. These beatings would last anything from five to ten minutes, I started holding in the tears and did not cry any more as I did not want him to see how much I was hurting inside.

It was very difficult to get started on this chapter. Dad passed away on May 20th 2009. We never had much of a father daughter relationship. I have also become a born-again Christian and have had lots of personal battles within myself about forgiving and letting go. That year (2010) I was forced to look at these issues head-on and Dad's death had a direct Impact on them.

Dad (May 2009-present)

Present

I recently had to look at my relationship with my dad as it has an influence on how I interact with men and my relationships with men. Because my dad never acknowledged me as a beautiful daughter and cherished me as one, I never felt worthy to be with any man. I chose poor partners that treated me badly and controlled me in some way or another and ended up changing to what they wanted me to become. This patterned continued until I was a grown young woman, attending college. I was dating a muslim guy during my second first year at Teacher's College, he was lovely, He did not even try to make me do stuff I did not want to you know, some fumbling and kissing and steamy feelings, but nothing more, he was respectful in that sense. One day I came home after lying to my parents that I went studying at a friends' after church and came home. Mum knew something was up, and threw Holy Water down our footpath as she said she does not want any Muslim Filth near her home. Dad got me to their room, asked me all sorts of questions and because I gave him the silent treatment, he got me to undress and sit naked in a corner as he then humiliated me. I guess he wanted to check if I was pregnant, I felt so ashamed and worthless, I guess now I knew I really hated him even more for not being a real dad to me and now he is embarrassing me and my mum did not even come to make him stop this. What kind of sick, twisted Christian gets his daughter to undress and then make her sit naked on the floor because she did not tell him what she got up to with a Muslim boy???

And the irony is that the Muslim boy was more than some of the Christian boys in all those respects as he did not want me to take my clothes off and have sex with him.

I dreaded going home to see dad and refused to go home as there was a Residential weekend for Counselling Course I HAD TO ATTEND AND I KIND OF WANTED TO USE IT TO STOP ME FROM GOING HOME (I really did not want to say goodbye to dad as he was such a mean dad to me after all and I felt I did not owe him anything). My friend said to me: "Go and say goodbye to your dad otherwise you will always regret it . . ."

I went and actually felt sorry for him as he was reduced to a shell of what he was . . . I arrived on the Saturday and dad passed away on the Wednesday the 20th on my wee (Scottish for "little") niece Lindy's birthday. I was the last person to be with him. Now South Africans call that "Blessed". If you were the last person to see your parents alive. My friend Tersia was the last person to be with her mum when she died. We are both "Blessed" according to Priscilla (Tersia's older sister).

Life or No Life (1972-1986)

My Primary school days were filled with visions of lines of children to the bathroom to brush our teeth and wash our faces.

First Year (Sub A) I had a lovely teacher called Miss P, who was lovely and who I adored.

I was sick one day, I think I had pickled fish in a tin and I was coming down with a virus or something to that effect. I cleaned up my sick and sat back down on the carpet, I had no thoughts of going home at all.

The teacher always used that story afterward to the rest of the class to show them that it was okay to stay in school after a little accident sometimes and I guess I felt special that she remembered that and I sure as hell did not receive any recognition from my parents so anything from another adult was great.

I did not know any better either as in our family no big fuss was made over you if you were sick. You would get your medicine and that was it, no big deal. No crying, no fuss, just get on with it and get over it. The rest of Primary School was fairly happy, I had my" wee" (wee means small in the Scottish language) gang of friends and if I did not have anybody to play with, I had my brothers and my sister was around too. The wetting episodes carried on all the way through to all of primary school and I was quite an anxious child.

After attending George Schmidt Moravian Primary School up to standard 3 (aged 8years old),about halfway through the school year we got moved to Frank Joubert Primary School in Korsten (a different coloured suburb in Port Elizabeth). The school was near Ouma Betty and Oupa Ben's house which meant we had to go wait there after school till Mum and Dad got home from work to pick us up.

I made new friends in this school and they soon found out that I wet myself. My friends covered for me when I was in a teacher's class that I did not feel safe enough to go and ask If I could leave the room or made me feel nervous in any way. To the frustration of the teachers I cried easily for silly little things—if I got the wrong page of maths or got the words spelt wrong or any minor mistake a normal child would brush off, I would react so strangely I think they thought I was a bit "Weird". Plus there was also the fact that I was new, and they did not know me well enough to know whether this was how I was or not. I started taking a spare set of clothes to school to change into. At this point I started stealing thing s from the other children's bags when I went out to toilet, first it was their lunch, then sweets, new toys. I thought because I went to Confession at the church on Saturdays, it was okay, I said my Hail Mary's and Our Fathers, but it never felt okay.

I felt bad when the children got upset when they found out their stuff were missing.

Sometimes I took stuff from my aunt's bags too, lipstick, coins sweets and silly little trinkets like pens, pretty hairpins and hair bobbles.

Weekends we went to Ouma Betty's as mum had to work and it seemed Dad had a job to go to. My unmarried aunts lived with Ouma Betty and Oupa Ben (this was quite common for children to live at their parents house until they get married or move out).One of my aunt's was a school teacher and she always had lovely nail polish, lipstick, jewellery and high heels, all a girl could wish for and dream of really. She let me play with all these things with no fuss whatsoever and I always thought this was great as my Mum did not allow us to touch any of her stuff at all. She also left her purse lying about as she was often in party mode when her other teacher pals (pals are Scottish slang for friends) came round and they had "good times" in her room. Ouma Betty called it, "The Pleasure Boat". One Saturday morning, I found myself raiding her for 50cent pieces and 20 cents pieces in order not to look so obvious that some money was missing. I would hide it in my shoes in case my clothes pockets would get searched. One Saturday mornings, while I was checking my loot, I had my shoe off and one of my other aunts (a younger one) walked in on me and caught me red handed. She called my schoolteacher aunt and Ouma Betty and asked me why I did it and also gave me a good talking to. If that was not bad enough and embarrassing enough, they phoned Mum and when she came to pick us up, I got the beating of a lifetime. I just took it and cried silently inside because I did not want them to see how ashamed, hurt and guilty I felt. I just wanted to be hugged and told it was going to be all right.

My mum's older sister was an Indian looking, smooth-skinned, dimpled face with soft silky wavy jet black hair, lived in a nearby neighbourhood. She had lots of children (my cousins). One of her daughters has the same birthday as mine and we got on really well. She is older than I am 5 years or so.

She used to bring me presents and always phoned me on my birthdays.

This particular aunt also left her purse out and I stole from her too, silver coins to start with mostly; 20 cents, 50 cents and later on R1 coins and even sometimes R5 notes too. I loved going to their house as we were allowed to play out in the streets with our cousins and their friends. Next door to my aunt lived a girl my age who was very streetwise and she seemed to take a shine to me (she liked me). I thought no one liked me and I was really the opposite of her, she was fair with light blue-green eyes, blonde hair and very confident and boy could she swear!!! Myself on the other hand was ugly, skinny, not very confident and have totally nothing to offer and extremely shy. I could not figure this one out AS we were total opposites, but I LOVED SPENDING TIME WITH HER. I did not steal from her mum and dad. We would spend time together eating sweets, listening to music in her room, when we got fed up doing that, we would patrol the streets.

Everyone knew her and this was absolutely great to be with someone who was so popular as I never was popular quite the opposite, I would almost fade away and become invisible.

Later I moved on to High School a school called St Thomas Secondary School. It was interesting and I made plenty of good friends, I stayed away from boys though and they disgusted me for some reason. Kissing, I thought was the most Yucky thing to do and anything else I could not even think about. The school used to be a Catholic school, but it was not anymore, but you were allowed to attend Mass at the Church across the road (St Martin De Porres) on significant days like Ash Wednesday, Ascension Thursday and other saint days or feast days.

At high school I stole less, but I did steal a little embroidered pouch from the Needlework and Craft cupboard while we were helping the teacher get ready for the external examiner coming in and we also getting our pieces together for external inspection and grading. I found this big, brown envelope at the back of the cupboard with some other knitted and crochet items. Normally I would ask first if I could have it, but this day I took it and put it into my school bag.

I took it to school the next day and started using it as a pencil case in all the classes. Later in the week, while we were in the Needlework Lesson, I had the embroidered pouch on my desk, the teacher noticed it and asked me: "Where did you get that, I have been looking everywhere for it? It is one of the Standard eight's final piece for examination." She was getting redder and redder as she spoke to me. I replied:"I found it in the cupboard while I was clearing out stuff the other day."

She told me that she had to take me Principal's office as I stole the pouch. MY friends all protested on my behalf as I never do stuff like that and that I admitted I took it and that she should let it go, but the teacher would not listen to any of them. At The end of that day in my accountancy lesson we had a visit from the Principal himself and he said: "Can I see Jacintha Canary please about the pouch you took?" "My spirit died that day, imagine that after having never been in trouble, now I was on my way to the Principal's office and probably gona be asked to leave school."

I bet Mum would be told and was waiting for me in his office, my heart sank to my toes.

Mum was waiting in the Principal's Office, her face looked so tired and the expression of disappointment was too much for me to handle. The principal asked me: "Do you realise what you have done?" I replied: "Yes, I am sorry, I won't do that again."

I had to go back home with Mum and she did not say a word on the way home. I wonder what she thought "what a disappointment, she wets the bed, now she steals in school too." I did not get a beating either. That night I wet the bed, again and the whole week thereafter.

My friends all stuck op for me and assured me that the Principal and Needlework Teacher were way too hard on me and they made sure the rest of the class never teased me about it either. I stopped stealing from Mum for a while after that, I could not get the thought out of my head that she had to get the phone call at work and then had to tell her boss what exactly????"My daughter is a thief, I have to go to the school and go see the Principal. May I have permission to leave? "

I found comfort in food instead, eating to fill the hole of empty hurt, loss, guilt, shame and sadness. I ate everything and anything and did not know when to stop. I hid it in my nightdress, in my cupboard, in my drawer and in any space I could find.

Best Friend (1986-present)

One of my best friends at high school was called Janice, she was beautiful with lovely brown skin, beautiful brown eyes, a soft voice, hair always made in a lovely style, extremely kind, thoughtful and sure of herself. I guess in one way she was all the qualities I wished I had all rolled into one, neat package. Janice had two brothers, both of them younger than her, her mum was a senior teacher at a Primary School and her dad worked in a car manufacturer's in Port Elizabeth. Her mum dropped her off every morning and came to collect them at the end of the school day. Sometimes her mum was late and I would stay with her till her mum came. We would walk around the school during break times, share and swap lunches and just hang out having girl chats. She also loved sewing even though she was a braniac (loved Maths and Physics, Accountancy (You know number subjects). Sometimes we would find an empty class and sew our items. I visited Janice's house and we baked biscuits, cakes, pies and even tried cooking stews and what not. (it was great fun going to Her place). Later on after our folks (parents) got to know each other we got to have sleepovers because they kind of trusted us to be sensible. I mostly went to Janice's house as I did not really like being at my house, because my sister and I shared a room so that meant that we were never really alone.

Janice's mum was very loving and loved giving us hugs all the time (so unlike my mum), she was bubbly, funny and very sophisticated. Janice's dad was very funny, loved pinching my nose and adored his daughter and treated her like a princess. When he came home from work, he would kiss us both and made us laugh with some funny comment or story. He would always compliment his wife's food and thanked us for making him cups of tea. This was so different from our household. Breakfast, lunch and dinners were formal occasions where we all sat down at the table, our manners would be corrected, our handling of the cutlery and our chewing and sound effects (loud noises while eating or drinking) too. It was a solid friendship with Janice and I still can't believe we are still friends, I mean what did I have to offer her? I was ugly, poor, not got a big house like hers and I did not have much confidence. At the sleepovers I even wet the bed at Janice's house (how embarrassing??), but her mum and dad did not make a big deal. They just told me to put the wet bedding in the bathroom and change the bedding with fresh bedding and maybe have no drinks after 7pm at nights. This was so strange, no criticism, sarcasm, shouting and comments about my laziness to get up and go to the bathroom at night time.

After completion of High School we went on summer holiday to my cousin's (on Dad's side) in Knysna for a week and then we went to Janice's cousin's place in the Karoo, which was about a two hour journey inland. The summers were dry and the winters dry and cold. Their place was a big, wonderful,5 bed roomed magnificent piece of art. It had two seperate TV rooms, a large kitchen with a Pantry, a large dining room with an Oak set, large oval table that seated 12. They had a maid that came in everyday and all we had to do was feed the little ones at breakfast times and lunch times (that varied as most of the time the little ones played away and the maid gave them whatever they needed when they were hungry. Sometimes the maid would give the little ones their breakfast especially if she knew were out late the previous evening . . . Gosh I had never had that much freedom and space, let alone time to go clubbing Wednesdays, some Thursdays, Fridays and even some Saturdays and sometimes midnight till 4:00am the next day, this was utter heaven.

Wednesdays was ladies night which meant all ladies (girls) got in from 7pm for free and the guys would be allowed in around 9pm at a charge.

That summer of 1989 I met a lovely young man who was older than me by five years (A student doctor in his fourth year at well known University in Cape Town. He was 21 and I was 17 and a half. His name was Conrad O'Brein. I met him by chance when we went to visit some relatives of Janice's cousin and I did not pay much attention to him as I was hooked on the green-eyed specimen who looked like a player and would never look at me in a million years. I was right because every other woman thought the same and he knew it too . . . . So Conrad was not the most attractive, but he was a gentleman with brains . . . . I mean come on he was studying medicine (I always fancied being the wife of top lawyer, psychologist, dentist or doctor. Well a girl's got to have dreams . . . although later on I quite liked the idea of being on my own with no man and no attachments thank you very much after I found out all this dating stuff is not that great after all.

He took me for drives after the Disco's and we kissed and did some fumbling above the navel . . . mum always said above the navel or else you will get pregnant and we were told not to bother coming home if we were to fall pregnant and these words kept ringing in the back of my head at all times when I was getting hot and bothered with Conrad in the car.

This guy must have thought I was way too "priss", but never said so. He was a gentleman and respected my wishes, but he did teach me a few things about feet and their place for passion . . . . I was however conscious of my smelly, dusty feet so before closing time, I would nip to the bathroom, wash and rub it with lovely lotion (a girl has to make an effort you know).

After that summer the romance continued and we remained in contact, this suited me fine as I love writing, I sprayed the letters with my perfume so that they could remind him of me. Dad did not approve, mum was chuffed that he was a doctor or soon to be. Status points were very important in the coloured community along with your looks, the lighter you are the better your chances, and the straighter and smoother your hair.

He told me that I was beautiful on a regular basis and he adored my frizzy curls dad wanted me to straighten all the time. He sent me teddy bears and flowers for Valentines. Once he sent me a mysterious bouquet before he came down to see me saying "A frizzy for the flowers" (a dozen red roses). I ignored it, but that night he arrived at my door and my hair was in a French Plait, Needless to say I dashed into the bathroom, washed my hair and frizzed it!(adding lots of conditioner and styling creams courtesy of Wella and Lo'real. He was so Romantic. Mum loved him straight away and said he had great manners, I loved his torn jeans (it had holes at the knees and a little bit below the derriere and I loved placing my fingers through them to tickle his legs. Dad was his usual grumpy self and did not make much conversation and asked all the FBI questions about Conrad and his family.

I got to see him for that whole weekend, it was great and even better still Janice was down from her Technikon so I got to hang out with my two closest people in my life!!!

We spent lots of time just hugging, kissing and being close. He was very protective over me and just treated me well and spoiling me with lovely gifts. When he left he asked me to come and see him in Graaff-Reinett in April so I said I would have to ask my folks permission.

I knew mum might consider it and dad would definitely say NO.

So I lied and told them I was going to a retreat with the nuns for a whole week in Port Elizabeth.

They bought it!!!

I travelled by taxi so I had to get to Ouma Betty's, stayed overnight then caught the next early taxi to Graaff-Reinett. I was very nervous, but also excited to see Conrad again after a long three months. I stayed at his sister's friend's house as we could not live together or sleep together that was not the done thing in the community or society for that matter. Unmarried young men and women do not live together (1990). I had a lovely time, but I was s_____g myself in case anyone found out My parents did not know where I was really . . . . Mum phoned to the house on the Thursday and asked "where are you and what are you doing there and why did you n ot go to the retreat?" I was found out and I had to return as soon as possible. It was actually a relief and I realised I am not ready for all that commitment stuff and I was maybe too young, an older girl would just be able to make her own way there and back, no questions asked but because I was just 18 and still living with my parents and not classed as an adult until I am 21 my hopes did not look that great. Poor Conrad I got him into the mess as well, because now my dad thought that he put me up to it and that I was sleeping with him (which I was not). I got a lift with Conrad's family friends a stern faced man that reminded me of my dad and after I told him my story he gave me a piece of his mind and said nothing more after that, so it was so long, silent, thinking Oh S__t what next?

Dad was out in the garden when we finally arrived in Port Elizabeth, I said my thank you and goodbye and paid the gentleman. I went in past dad, he did not say much and he did not follow me in to the house like usual when he has something to say or reprimand me for.

I went to my room, my oldest brother Nathaniel came in to say Hi and see how I was doing. (he was always very protective over me too). We chatted for a while, I think my oldest sister was in the kitchen. I went out into the garden and told my dad "Ek is jammer." Direct translation—"I am sorry." Dad told me how he had been at church and he was chatting to one of the deacons and told him I was a retreat, when the deacon told him there was no retreats that weekend." I guess he must have felt quite proud that I was still involved with the church life.

Dad then asked the dreaded question: "Why did you lie to me?" I said: "you would have said no anyway so I thought that you would say yes to the retreat and that is what happened." Dad went quiet when he was unhappy and that is what happened. Mum did not say much either and shook her head. Conrad phoned that evening and dad was going off so my brother stepped in and took the phone off him, a courageous thing to do. We kept our long distance relationship going even though dad did his occasional, "get of the phone" routine shouts.

The summer holiday I went back to Graaff-Reinett with Janice, that would be my last one. One night Conrad picked me up and took me to another place far up in the mountains, he wanted to show me something different I guess. When we got there, there were four white youths and immediately I felt . . . we should go and get out of there as they were up to no good.

While we were parking one of them came up to the car and asked: "Wat soek jy hier hotnot?" (hotnot is a derogatory term a white person uses for a coloured).Really very condescending and aggressive. Conrad said: "Niks nie." (nothing much) I told him to tell the guy we were looking for someone and we should go, but before he could do that the guy swung a punch at his face. Conrad wanted to get out of the car and punch the guy back. This time I firmly told him: "LET'S GO NOW!", in no UNCERTAIN TERMS. Through the corner of my eye I could see the guy motioning his buddies to come and join us, I just thought: "No ways, they are going to beat us up, rape me and what else. Having been sexually abused I was not going to get messed with by nobody." We left much against Conrad's wishes I think, but thank goodness he listened at the time. He drove down to the club to get his mates, drop me off and return I guess to give those guys a good beating. I stayed with Janice AND the girls, a little shook up. A long while later, the guys returned, they did not find them and I was relieved because this could have gotten ugly and turn into a race thing, and we knew who would get the blame (The coloured guys). Conrad was never the same after that, I reassured him that he did nothing wrong and I still thought of him as my gentleman and hero.

A couple of months later we split up, he found someone older and I was getting attention from a second year male student. I still heard about him through the grapevine.

College (January 1990- November 1993)

....

After High School I enrolled into Teacher's College at Dower Training College in Port Elizabeth. This was recommended as one of the best for teacher training in South Africa. Really I did not want to be there, and did not attend the classes, needless to say I failed the first year.

I lied to my friends, but my mum told the the truth already, so when term re-started I had to join in with all the freshmen and re-sit through all the orientation days of the first term.

I was really angry most of the time and hung out with my second year mates. I did not cooperate much in the lessons and scowled most of the time, except in the history and language classes because these lecturers I actually liked because they knew their stuff.

I had a thing going with the bad boys because I was so full of S__t! That meant I got lots of special attention and privileges during break times and student get-togethers.

Class attendance was something I had to do second time round or else I could fail on attendance even if I passed my exams, so I made an effort.

My English lecturer decided to go on a Secondment halfway through the year and we got this retired, old teacher with a restless and roaming eye for beautiful young bodies and roaming hands. All the girls went to give him kisses and hugs when they met him in the corridor. This meant he would tick them as present even though they never turned up for some lessons, he would also keep their notes for them and give them pass marks for all their assignments and other little perks or ADDED EXTRAS . . . .

I DID NOT PARTICULARLY LIKE THIS AND DETESTED HIS SLEEZINESS. I SIDESTEPPED HIM WHEN HE WOULD LOOK LIKE HE WAS GOING TO EMBRACE ME AD I CERTAINLY DID NOT INTEND TO KISS SOME OLD DUDE WHO HAD NOTHING BETTER TO DO THAN WAX LYRICAL ABOUT HIS Teaching highlights and not do his work he was paid to do, because he was not getting enough attention from his family. This went on for a whole term, I watched all this and I thought enough is enough. I went to the rector (Whose son I dated in the past so I felt comfortable with him) and told him all this. I knew I was going to get a fail, I was expecting that. Not long after that he was asked to leave. I knew my lecture would return and my grades would go up to what they should be.

Much to the distress of the other girls, our professional, smart and dedicated lecturer returned who actually knew his subject matter. Phew!!!

For the next two years I kept my head down and actually enjoyed some of it, I got introduced to a freshman in my third year who played for the rugby team and he was the most well-built stud I have seen in a long time. I did not know what he was doing with me, but hey he was gentle and strong and I loved the fact that he was tall.

I sometimes snuck into the men's hostel to see him in his room . . . many times I got caught in the corridors when the vice—rector would be doing spot checks . . . .

I completed my teacher's training Diploma in 1993 and got a position in a small town near Grahamstown.

Past Relationships

When I graduated from Teacher's College I took the most faraway teaching job I could get in order to be away from home. I did not want to be at home near my parents as they were too controlling and I did not particularly get along with them. At that time I dated this guy who I met through my best friend Janice who was studying in Cape Town at one of the Technikons up there. This guy was studying at The University of Western Cape at the time. During holiday times we would go clubbing a lot, Janice and I as we both loved dancing. I was not on the lookout for anybody at the time, I had a short thing with one of the second year students at College, but he too was a gentleman and we only kissed and cuddled and did not get any further than that. I kind of liked this guy because he had a gentleness about him, he drank a little too much, but hey at least he did not look like he was a beater and he was not critical at all. We went out to the movies a couple of times and he took me for a meal once, but that was it. Sometimes he would forget to turn up and I would wait up for him, not call him to ask if he forgot, but after a few times I did call and of course he did not pick up his phone then, Mum told me to go out with my friends and not wait up any more (she did not say he was no good, but I guess she was looking out for me). He kept in touch in his own way and always took me and Janice to the club and home and then we would kiss and you know what . . . but only on these nights, I was beginning to think there is something wrong with me.

I moved away after qualifying from Teacher's College and started teaching and then I kept in contact with him, but he never responded much and he forgot my birthday for the second time, so I wrote him a letter to tell him it was over and I wished him well for his future as he did not seem to have the time to have a relationship.

I finished in Fort Beaufort and moved up to Umtata (Transkei, Nelson Mandela's Homeland).

This was a pre-dominantly black city and the first words my mum told me was that I am going to get shot and Black people are not to be trusted. I found this all very re-assuring as I wanted to be rebellious and do things that would go against their grain. I hooked up with a former class mate from college as she was the one who got in touch with me about the position.

This was great, we were a bunch of young graduates fresh from College most of us in our first or second year of teaching. We lived in a big three bed roomed house in a prominent area near the city centre attractions. There was not much in the way of shopping complexes, just one complex, no movies or cinema and no beach or other form of usual entertainment. We went to church most Sundays and the other times we hung out together spending time cooking new recipes, travelling to beach resorts once a month or going to East London where one of my roommates were from. This was very exciting as we then got to go to the clubs there, spent all our hard earned money on ridiculous amounts of clothes and gadgets. I did not want to go home so I only went home at the long school holidays. I had no particular interest in any guys at this point either as I needed time to get over this guy who never seemed to have time for me so men were not a priority and as I was used to my own company many Saturdays when the rest of the housemates went out, I was quite happy cooking, baking biscuits and tidying up I suppose as I was used to doing that at mum's house on Saturdays. I got bored with the shopping, clubbing routine and I saw it as a waste of money as I was not into drinking all that much.

I kept myself busy with lesson preparation and volunteered my skills at the Primary School in the afternoons during the week. In my second year of teaching at the Primary School, this new male teacher started at the school and he became like the second in charge at the school. He was not particularly good-looking or interesting, but something about how he carried himself caught my attention. He was way older than me, in his forties and I was 23. I started making time to be around him and we had some interesting debates around politics, religion and society which I found highly entertaining. At last I thought someone who can keep me interested and not some stupid boyfriend trying to impress me with cool clothes, fast cars and how much he can drink and show off in front of his mates. I was so sick of them and did not see how girls could find those guys attractive or even interesting, I thought if you have no thinking power than I definitely do not want anything to do with you at all. He asked me out a couple of times and we became an item. He picked my housemate and I up in the morning and dropped us off after school, this was great!!!

I fell pregnant soon after we started dating, but he did not want the baby, I was torn because I was a Catholic and I would be taking a life. I was not even scared of what my Mum would say if I told her. I was prepared for that speech and I was prepared to be single mum, what I wasn't prepared for was this man telling me that he wants me and not the baby. His reasoning behind it was that he had a child already and was divorced and that he just did not want any kids. I saw a different side to him which I did not like and I was beginning to go off him very fast, but he would not leave me alone. He even offered to pay for the abortion on his medical aid.

I had the abortion and I never told my mum or my parents. Instead I went to confession and confessed that I killed a baby and got my penance of twenty Hail Mary's and ten Our Fathers. (I am not wanting to portray the Catholic Faith in a negative light in any way so please take this within my context and so not generalise as each case is different). I could not believe that this was it and I plagued myself with guilt and could not forget what I have done. I went to my housemate's one holiday and we went to a fortune teller (she read our tea leaves and this was my first encounter with fortune telling. This was a supposedly a good experience, but I felt my stomach churn all the way there and back and I could not let go so I felt so bad about that, that I went to confession at the Catholic Church and the priest there made me feel so bad, dirty, cheap and no-good at all.

During that time I became really depressed and withdrew from all activities, I would go to school, come home, go to my room and listen to music or just lie there and pretend to read if any of my roommates came in. I felt homesick, but I could never get myself to tell my parents, God was the only one who knew about the abortion and sexual abuse. I thought the sexual abuse was the better news of the two that my folks could cope with and I never told them about the abortion, I thought that it would kill my mum. I was a big sinner, full stop and no amount of Hail Mary's and Our Fathers would ever rid me of my guilt for killing a little boy Foetus.

I went for confession with this lovely old, Swedish father and Still to this day I have difficulty forgiving myself, I have come through this, but it is difficult and painful to deal with even to this day.

It was a boy and he would have been born on the 7th of December 1996. I named him Daniel (brave one). The 7th Of December is a special date that stays in my mind as he will always be in my heart. I have crying days, sad days, battles with God about him forgiving me and me still not being able to forgive myself. I am learning to accept God's total forgiveness, I am a murderer and God still loves me, I still find this difficult to understand, but I am getting better at that too.

When I ended with this man, I could not get him to understand that I did not want anything to do with him anymore. One day he drove me out of town and threatened to kill me as he knew somebody else was showing an interest in me. I do not know how I got home that day, but I was praying silent prayers of help to God. Till this day I do not know how I got back to home, but after that I never went anywhere without my friend even the bathroom or up to the office to speak with the secretary or headmistress. Soon after that he got a promotion at another prestigious private school to join the management team.

I started having lots of nightmares and strange dreams of feeling really scared and woke up crying like a little girl in the middle of the night. I could not shake the feeling of being uncomfortable around men and I did not have periods, but instead I had these excruciating pains in my female organs. I went to my local doctor who then referred me to a gynaecologist and obstetrician. He was a lovely, kind man who discovered that I had ovarian cysts and he gave me some treatments for the cysts to go away. I kept going back though for check-ups and one day whilst in his surgery I told him about my dreams. He sat quietly and listened until I finished and he asked me about my scary dreams and about my childhood. Up until then I thought I had a happy childhood, (okay I know, my parents were a bit strict and all and a tad controlling, but they loved us in their own way, Just did not express it enough). I remembered some upset about the man who used to touch me and made me do some strange things with his penis at around the age of 9 and a half ten. He called it sexual abuse. He also told me to have some time off school and that also think about telling my parents. "No way!", I said, "I could never tell my parents they won't believe me!" He said he still thought I should think about it and when I do, he will refer me to a good Psychiatrist in Port Elizabeth as I will need some support to get through this and work through the issues relating to the sexual abuse. I took time off from school to think and in that time I kind of spent some time with this Scottish guy who came round our house most days to visit our housemate. (In a friendly way as I did not want anything to do with guys). I did not pay much attention at first, but then I kind of noticed the lovely blue-green eyes, the long blonde hair and the lovely smile. Secretly I thought (mmmmmm not bad for a white dude, but not for me right now thank you very much, being a Catholic girl and all, I know after the last mess and the abortion . . . .). My parents will kill me if I come home with A WHITE DUDE LET ALONE A FOREIGN ONE AT THAT!!!! I COULD JUST HEAR MY DAD'S RESPONSE: "WHAT IS WRONG WITH YOU? YOU KNOW IT CAN'T WORK. What will your kids be?"

He turned out to be a good laugh and he made me smile a lot more than I have been since the break-up with the older deputy head. We stayed friends for a while as I told him the sex-thing won't work for me just now, and he said: "No pressure". I thought, (great a guy who listens and understands to a woman).

To test his ball strength, I told him quite early on about the sexual abuse, actually I wanted to scare him off and wanted to make him run as far as the hills. I really did not feel up to any kind of relationship and then on the other hand I wanted him to say, "it's okay, everything will be just fine, I will take care of you, which he did so I was a bit S_____D. He stuck around and I kind of let him grow on me . . . .

This was new and totally different to any other guy experiences I had since the three lovely guys I had after high school, college and teaching as a professional. He seemed really nice, a bit on the stingy side, he did not like to part with his money and did not treat me with gifts, meals out and other stuff most coloured guys do to impress and keep their woman, and I thought sure a bit different and because I did not want to go out anyway in case I bumped into Mr. Abortion I kind of overlooked it even though my girlfriends pointed it out on a few occasions that he was a tad selfish . . . . I thought, so what I kind of like him so we will see what happens and he was definitely not like any other guys.

I convinced myself that he must be a really genuine guy after all.

A week later, I went home to go and tell my parents about the sexual abuse. My mum's response was," I knew there was something very wrong as You always acted very strange". My dad's response was, "What did he give you?". I replied, "money, sometimes sweets" to which my dad said, "You were nothing but a prostitute!". Mum shouted at him and I ran off somewhere to my friend's house. (Carmen who lived round the corner from us and I knew she would listen and understand and console me) secretly I thought all parents were messed up because, why did they never get their children? These words of dad, however stuck around in my head for a long time all through most of my adult life. Not exactly the comforting words you would like to hear after you have just told your folks you have been messed around by an adult you were told to trust. Not exactly the words you want to hear at a vulnerable time in your life where you just took a month or two to get the courage together to open up.

Fortunately Mum shouted at him to "S__t up!"

That night we had a family gathering, with my parents, brothers and myself. My parents did not think my sister and her husband could be privy to this information as they were not flavour of the month because of family stuff that was happening at their wedding.

We were told by my parents that nobody should know and this news about my sexual abuse should stay within the family, your sister is not to know as she might tell her husband and he in turn might tell his family. This was not to be challenged and that was the last time it would be discussed ever, in the closet and there it will stay.

I stayed at home for a month after that to recover and I received sessions with a great Psychiatrist, then I returned to Umtata for a while and then went back down to resume my sessions with the psychiatrist.

Upon return from the last visit home, I received a phone call from my headmaster and he informed me that I would not have a job to come back to as I have been off for longer than my contract stipulated and my notice money would be paid into my bank account. I tried to fight the unfair dismissal, but gave up as my energy levels were low and I felt I had to concentrate on getting better.

Wedding Bells from Scotland (September 1996- December 1996)

This was yet another setback and a fight I did not have energy to fight so I went to the school with My Scottish boyfriend (yes things have progressed quite a bit by then) he offered to accompany me and I went to collect my things. I stopped by the headmaster's office and said my piece and the dude also added his piece in a polite manner. Then I thanked him and wished him well as mum always told us to wish people well, especially if they are ill mannered and not so polite. (I did not always get this one cheek and offer the other cheek but I guess mum knew and Now as a Christian I know that all is not always as it seems and by praying for people especially if they are treating you badly you need to pray even more)

I lived with the dude at his place for a while, because I could not afford rent as well or I had to go back to my folks' place.

Three months later I asked him to marry me, to test his loyalty and also I wanted to end the relationship because it was getting too comfortable And that stage I always think, "Oh S__t!" this is getting too close and I need out. He accepted. I thought to myself, "once he has met dad he will most definitely change his mind!"

I took him to meet my parents during the September break.

Mum loved him of course. Dad did not make any secret of his feelings towards whites.

You see dad lived in a white neighbourhood, but then they got re-classified as coloured and got kicked out to the coloured suburbs and he never got over this. He was very bitter about that and I guessed slowly destroyed him from the inside harbouring all that bitterness and resentment.

At nights we said evening prayers we all had to attend whether you believed in God or not, that was a house rule. Dad said the evening prayers in Afrikaans in order to exclude my boyfriend.

I thought this was very rude and I told my dad that, he did not say anything to that or change the way he said prayers (English in stead of Afrikaans).

Later on my boyfriend felt, maybe we needed to sit my folks down and tell them his intentions are honourable and that he was here to stay. We did that one day, 'whoah', I still do not know where that came from as I kept communicating with dad to a minimum.

Things changed a little since that frank conversation with my parents and dad said evening prayers in English, sometimes he would revert to Afrikaans every so often.

We got married the lovely Scotsman and I on the 14th of December 1996 in my hometown of Port Elizabeth. It was funny though because I caught the bouquet at my sister's wedding the year before . . . now I do not believe in all that because the guy I was seeing had no thoughts about marriage and I knew we would not go far as he was way too into his friends and he always forgot my birthday . . . .

Eight of my boyfriend's family members came over to join us on our wedding day. Because it was such a small attendance from my husband's side we kept my family attendance to a minimum only friends and close family was invited to the reception afterwards, but most people attended the Church part and we had a barbecue on the Sunday for the people who could not attend the reception.

I know, very Western, a lot of unhappy people and gossip went round I am sure, but it was better that way.

The newly acquired in-laws spent Christmas and New Year in South Africa.

My mother-in-law wanted to be called by her first name. That was not what we did in South Africa as you call your mum and dad-in-law (Mum and dad) as you gain a second set of parents so to speak.

This took some time of getting used to as I kept thinking I was being rude calling an adult by their first name as we were not brought up to do that. All adults should be addressed as aunty or uncle, mrs, mr, father, pastor and that was the way it was drilled into us as coloured children with manners and respect.

Christmas we spent eating food and drinking some bubbly, wine, beers and whatever else people wanted. Mum cooked hers usual leg of lamb, a Cornish hen, salted beef (soutvleis), Ox tongue, a curry stew, beetroot salad, carrot and pineapple salad, cucumber salad, tomato salad, fridge tart and trifle and much much more (yummy, yummy). We did not have a tree and all the glitzy presents as we did not do big glitzy Christmases as we focused on Jesus's birth and togetherness with the family, food, more food, people coming over to eat desserts, samoosas, pies, savoury biscuits with cheese and tomato, anchovies and light sandwich fillers. It is an eating affair and a sense of being happy and merry and sharing with all the folks popping by that is how it goes down in the coloured neighbourhood.

We did not have a tree with any presents under it.

Later on all of us went to Transkei at Hole-in-the wall a holiday resort near Coffee Bay and we all spent time together. I learnt quite a bit about the family dynamics over that week.

My father-in-law almost drowned that week and I saw a new side to my sister-in-law that was not there the week before, I was beginning to wonder what else I did not know.

We went back to Port Elizabeth again for a short while and then we went up to Cape Town to celebrate New Year as well as go and explore some of the tourist attractions.

Looking back now, it was really a bad idea to honeymoon with the family as everybody has their own ideas of how they would like to spend their time and I realised that too late in the holiday.

The family went home and Shaun and I returned to Port Elizabeth. We then started the process of getting my visa to go abroad to The United Kingdom.

I had to go to Pretoria (Now Gauteng) to attend an interview with the British High Commission to verify whether this marriage was authentic or not and whether they would approve my visa application. The questions they asked still baffle me—"How long did you date?"; "Did you write love letters to each other?"; "What was the colour of the bridesmaid dress?"; "Why did you get married?" "What is the name of your Parish Priest that married you?"

Really I thought to myself, how will that tell them anything about me? I felt the questions were really nothing related to the visa application and I felt like saying that to them, but my husband said they might deny my application so I should just listen and answer the questions.

PART 2

Life in the UK (February 1997)

The visa was approved and we left South Africa on February the 26th 1997 and arrived in wet and grey London on the morning of 27th February 1997. This was not cool, I knew it would be cold, but the greyness, the closeness of the houses and the lack of space in the homes they called flats was something I struggled to adapt to, I missed the sunshine, waking up to the sun, walking bare feet wearing skirts, denim shorts, skirts, dresses, colourful t-shirts, my weird and wonderful neighbour's kids and being able to walk down the road to my sister's place, opening the pots and eating junk from her pantry and seeing my niece who was just 6months old at the time and really cute and huggy.

I missed home terribly and I phoned my mum every other day asking them what they were doing and eating and what the weather was like. I also told my mum; "I want to come home. "

Mum replied: "It's better there, you can make a new start and forget about all the stuff from the past."

I accepted it and said goodbye with lumps in my throat.

I decided to focus on getting a teaching job and started applying to Primary Schools as the dream of returning in five years and running our own business kept me focused.

My husband and I were very much in love and I thought; "yes, everything will be alright. Everything is possible if we stick together. I have a new family and my husband loves me more than I love myself."

We lived with my sister-in-law and her husband in the county of Surrey, they too were two newly weds themselves who got married the year before.

I had absolutely no intentions of getting close to my sister in-law as I saw in south Africa how she showed no respect for her parents so I did not really reach out to her or return her attempts to become friends.

I tried my best to fit in, but ultimately I went out less and less as there seemed to be a big focus on going to the pubs. I found this strange as in South Africa we all socialise in each others' homes, we cook good food, share company and drink in the house around the fire in summer and inside during Autumn and winter. This was their life and I did not see the point in spending your money on alcohol, getting drunk and then not even remembering who said what the next day?

The outside was cold due to the weather, the houses were cold . . . . I missed the warmth and social vibes of South Africa and the closeness of touching and hugging as we are an affectionate bunch. (I missed that)

The job applications did not go so well either as all the primary schools wanted people with experience of the British curriculum. I joined a Recruitment Agency and did what they call supply teaching. If a school phones up the agency calls you and you have to go and teach there at the school. It could be a day, two days a week and at times a term or two.

I did not like this as I missed the stability of going to a school, getting to know the children and knowing their parents. I did not like going from school to school, not knowing what to say and people not understanding my South African accent and me not understanding the British accent. I thought everybody spoke good spoken English like we were taught in schools from the age of five. These people did not speak the English we were taught, sometimes they missed letters; like Alwhite instead of all right? In-it in stead of isn't it. People hardly smiled back at you and would ask you: "What you looking at?"

I ended up in inner city schools of London, in the surrounding areas like Purley, Croydon, Sydenham, Islington. Most of the children were tough, defensive, hardly listened and the question of manners were a dying trait, there were some well behaved ones, but they were in the minority.

Being a Catholic I got to teach at some Catholic schools and some of them asked me back as the children seemed to like me. Don't get me wrong some Catholic schools also had difficult classes, but there was a familiarity with knowing what to expect, growing up as a Catholic.

In the meantime I was still applying for jobs as a regular teacher as I wished for my own class, but I only reached the interview stage and never got hired. I did not know that I could ask for feedback and some schools gave me feedback and some did not.

That really was hard to swallow as I regarded myself as a great teacher and my references reflected that. I guess the depression started then, but I did notice the signs.

A Break in Edinburgh, Scotland (April 1997)

During The Easter Break we went up to Edinburgh in Scotland to see my mother-in-law and father in-law. His mum and dad arranged a "wee" (small) party in order to meet the family. This was lovely and I felt part of a family for a few moments and the depression seemed to be far away during that break.

We also made an effort to meet my husband's friends and we were cooking a meal for one of his closest friends one afternoon and my husband and I seemed to be arguing over the smallest thing and I have not seen this side of him and I struggled to understand what I have done to make him behave like this. One day I felt really guilty for causing him to be so bad-mooded and I decided to take an overdose of his mum's sleeping tablets. When I told him what I had done he just laughed and told me: "You are f_____g joking, I do not believe you." He carried on with cooking and ignored me, at that moment his parents walked in coming home from work, he told his mum and she asked me; "Did you take the tablets?" I replied: "yes I did." My husband did not come with to the hospital, I remember getting into the car with my mother-in-law and father-in-law and my mother-in-law saying; "keep your eyes open and stay awake."

My husband and I was fighting every day, I needed support as I gave him support and understanding in South Africa when My father was being unsympathetic, selfish and inconsiderate by praying and speaking in Afrikaans around my husband. I did not understand this "I do not care attitude" and "just get on with things as you are not in South Africa now and stop depending on me." He changed from this all protective "I love you and I will always be there for you, hugging and supportive husband" to this grumpy, bad-tempered and swearing man who stayed in bed most days who did not want to get up till around midday. I was an early riser so I was excited to go and see the city. I started feeling more and more lonely again feeling isolated and depressed.

The day I took the overdose, we were cooking because one of his closest friends was coming round to dinner and the last thing I remember was me asking about whether I am cutting the potatoes the right size or should I make them smaller. My husband's response was "I do not f_____g care!" This was happening a lot in the last few days which I was not used to being spoken to like that. Our way of speaking did not include swearing or any disrespectful talk, that was totally unacceptable.

I have had enough, I saw the tablets on the kitchen counter, took them to the bathroom and swallowed them there. . . .

I remember waking up in the Edinburgh Royal Infirmary hospital bed needing to do a poo, but the nurses held me down and would not let me get off the bed thinking I did not know what I meant. . . . I got up there and then did a poo in some bedpan-thing. Thank goodness otherwise it could have been a disaster and a smelly business at that. . . .

My husband was his loving self again and for a few weeks after that, he swore solemnly that he will love, protect and care for me. His parents decided it was best not to tell any of my family or friends not even my mum. I felt bad as I wanted my mum to know, but I did not tell her as I thought that they were probably right not to worry my mum with that.

My husband and I went up North to Aviemore where his Aunt had a static caravan and we had a lovely couple of days together. The fresh air was good and it brought us closer together.

It seems that getting away from things was a recurring theme in my life; away from South Africa to leave the Sexual Abuse, childhood emotional and physical abuse, a poor relationship with my dad and a lack of love for myself.

We went back down to London and moved out from My husband's sister and her husband to our own apartment/flat a week before my birthday 22nd April 1997.

At that point I was not really engaging much with my sister-in-law as I felt that we really did not get along however hard we tried. This was a great move towards freedom and I was excited at the thought of cooking my own food, watch television when I wanted (not that I watched much telly anyway). But with freedom comes new challenges, we were still drifting apart as a couple. My husband now went to visit his sister and his brother-in-law on his own. My husband told me to meet his sister in order to improve things so I did and I phoned her to meet up for a coffee somewhere, but she kept cancelling at the last minute, I left the door open. We drifted apart too.

My husband was doing better and managed to get hired for most of the week. He managed to secure a contract at a Secondary School in West Sussex, which meant we had to move again and I could then also apply for Primary teaching Jobs down that way.

I was thinking of home every day and I was very unhappy, the weather never seemed to be better . . .

My moods were low and my bubbly personality faded and faded at a fast rate. I was struggling and my daily chats with mum was the only thing that kept me going. My husband had enough to worry about so when he came home I would pretend things were alright, but at times when I tried to speak to him he would be dismissive and impatient as he wanted to watch football and have his beer and unwind.

I would then go to bed early and read my books. I also did not have a Catholic Church to go to and I missed that. From praying three times a day and attending church at least twice a week I had no connection with God apart from my daily Prayers and I was lacking that so much.

We were very far from the local Catholic Church as the buses only ran every two hours or so and we did not have much extra money as I could not secure a teaching position. I got a job as a Learning assistant and got paid a fraction of a teacher's wage. I started attending the local Church of England as I thought well it is the same God and He will understand that I cannot go to a Catholic Church because of financial constraints.

During the October Break my husband's parents came to visit us and bought us a few bits and pieces. It was lovely to have company and to have another woman to talk to.

A sofa bed so people have somewhere to sleep if they visited, a desk so my husband can do his writing. His mum also asked my husband whether she should buy us a chair each and I said, "Yes please", but my husband said, "No". We only needed one for him to sit at the desk. I was looking forward to having meals together as I was getting tired of sitting in front of the television eating our meals. You see in South Africa we sat around the table and ate together most times praying and talking about our days. I missed the togetherness of sitting round the table even just to chat and have a piece of cake. Mum cooked most of the times and during the week she would always bake a cake or a loaf of bread and the house was always smelling of yummy food as you walked through the door.

Not having that with my husband meant I would be sitting at the television and he would be on his chair which he reminded me of on a regular basis that it was his chair.

His mum also recommended that we move to Edinburgh, Scotland in December and apply for jobs up there and see if we could then get our own place after we saved up enough for a deposit.

I was getting really excited as his mum for all her "call me by my first name mentality", was a real family person and met up every Tuesday with her brothers and sisters. I thought this was great as that sounds like a "coloured thing to do" just we did it more often than once a week. My mother-in-law was an easy-going person and had lots of energy (this really amazed me that she always wanted to go on walks and explore the towns and local surroundings) and at times I wondered how they do that, as at times I was wiped out and really tired after all those walks and exploration trips.

Re-locating to Edinburgh (December 1997)

. . . .

We decided after long chats that we should give Scotland a go as we were not securing permanent jobs and we were not saving anything as we originally planned and I was missing home and family times. My husband thought that I could meet up with the family in Scotland as I was missing my family as his mum met up with her brothers and sisters once a week and I liked the sound of that.

I could also start attending the local Catholic Church and I thought I could also get involved with the church activities like I did back home in South Africa. Things were really looking up. We hired a van and drove up to Edinburgh, Scotland on the 19th of December 1997.

The journey was long and tiring, but also insightful. I saw another side of my husband that I had not seen for a while. I mean, I knew he could be selfish at times, arrogant perhaps and a tad self-centred. (I want to use a more descriptive word, but I would like to honour my daughters' as they will be reading this when they are old enough)

On the journey I heard myself being addressed as b____h, Cow to name but a few. We made it to Edinburgh safely and alive. In South Africa they had this campaign (" Arrive Alive") due to the high number of road accidents so I guess it is a standing joke to arrive alive, but it was also filled with a seriousness as I have lost family members and friends to car accidents.

Life in Edinburgh was good; I had a place to call home, a "mum and dad" to greet in the mornings, sit down with and have meals, almost like back in South Africa.

I struggled to get teaching registration with The General Teaching Council of Scotland.

They granted me Conditional registration for three years on the condition that I complete another degree of my choice which I had to fund.

I completed one year of an Advanced Diploma in Special needs and then did not complete the second year for personal reasons. I was finding it very difficult again to manage and my depression got worse somehow, but I plodded on and the weather was really getting to me. I signed up for A Sexual Abuse Survivors Group which met on Mondays for three months and that seemed to help.

We were also thinking of starting a family, I think that got me thinking all sorts of thoughts: will I be good enough? What will I do if it was girls? I wished it could be boys so that they could not be abused like me. In my head I felt that if I could sort out those thoughts it would free me up to then deal with the pregnancies and it would be okay that way. I seemed to operate on a checklist of emotions and feelings and if it is ticked then it won't be of any significance at all later on. In the end I REALISED THAT IT WOULD BE OKAY as long as the baby was healthy considering that I had an abortion and that I could be having all sorts of complications.

Little did I know that one cannot control these feelings, thoughts and emotions surrounding the feelings of any childhood issues as they come and go like the waves and tides of the sea (unknowingly and uncontrollably).

In January 2000 at the beginning of the year I received a phone call from a head teacher asking me to come and see her about a job. A friend was up visiting from South Africa and my husband's friend was still on holiday so I asked him to take me there and my friend chummed along (went along for the ride and company really) and we went one bright Tuesday morning, I went in and she offered me the position as a primary teacher of a composite class P1/2/3 in a lovely village setting. This was great after all the temporary positions I now had my own class, things were looking up, Yay!!!!

The relationship with my husband was deteriorating again. Weekends we did not get out of the house till about midday as he was still in bed. I would be up at early, ready to go out, but I was not so sure about the city centre and very much wanted him to come along.

He on the other hand seemed to have interest in little things, I encouraged him to start coaching Basketball again as I know he missed it and it would get him out and about. I started meeting up with some teacher friends and their flatmates who I met through school, mostly from New Zealand, Australia, Canada, Ireland and England to name a few. We would meet up for coffees and hang out at weekends going to shows, movies and gigs at quirky pubs in town.

I signed up again for support for my sexual abuse from the GP (General Practitioner) surgery and received counselling again for a 3 month period.

During this time I then had to get to terms with feelings around my dad (Scottish father-in-law) and his dependency on alcohol. I noticed that the relationship between my mother and father-in-law was not as committed as I thought and began to notice similar patterns in our marriage.

I wanted out as a few words rang in my head that a Catholic Nun told me "If there are more worse than betters in the marriage, it is time to review. "I never quite thought" I got it' or understood it, till that time. I had a friend who had a flat in Stockbridge and asked her if I could crash at hers for a while until I figured out what next. She said it was okay.

My husband begged me to stay and promised that we could work things out. I stayed keeping in contact with my mum back home and my best friends in South Africa, Janice, Tersia, Scharmelle and Carmen.

Things improved for a short while. In 1999 things were great, we went to LA, San Francisco and it was fantastic. We saw some old friends from South Africa and I fell in love with the place. It reminded me a lot of my hometown's weather. Warm breezy, misty and windy all rolled into one day at times. We fell in love again that year. It was a year of many changes.

Mum was going to come over in the Christmas period to Scotland and I was so excited as then she could see me and maybe I could persuade her to come back and help out with the baby when we got round to having it in the near future.

I had an epileptic attack one saturday during the September break in town near the Portrait Gallery in Edinburgh's city centre during the September of that year, my in-laws were away on holiday so it was only my husband and I. I was admitted overnight.

I told my mum and she said it was the cold, but I had to go for a CAT scan just to make sure.

The scan showed up an abnormality of the frontal lobe, they also wanted me to go back for a follow-up appointment in July the following year. The specialist told me: "You always look like you have the world on your shoulders." I felt I had to make an effort to look happier and I guess the sexual abuse lingered within me, but I was really alone and missed home terribly especially now being my second winter. The depression came back to haunt me always in winter it seemed.

A Sudden Goodbye (November 1999)

I was focussing on getting mum the financial assistance to get her passport in order to come over and secretly convince her to stay here. Sadly it was not meant to be, mum died on the 29th of November of that year (1999) in South Africa.

It came as a real shock as the Saturday before then I told her I received my module of having passed my first year of the Advanced Diploma in Special Needs from The Open University. She was really happy for me. The good thing about having come to Scotland was that we could rebuild our troubled and difficult relationship. We were on the phone every other day catching up with stuff and we became friends and confidants, but I could not get myself to tell her about the abortion and the suicide attempt.

The funeral was two weeks later. My mother in law booked the tickets and my husband and I went, I wanted to stay for Christmas, but my husband thought no I had to get back to work.

I still struggle at my inability to say no, inside I am thinking "I want to stay and spend the summer with my family and friends.",but I do not say that out loud and give in to my husband's instructions. You see a death is a celebration of someone's life when they die, it is a time for the family and friends to remember the person and mourn and grieve with close ones where you all feel supported through this process before and after the funeral.

My husband reasoned that two weeks would be enough and he heavily cramped my style when we were there. Mum talked a lot about her funeral (while she was still alive) and how she wanted it to be so my sister and I made sure that she got the send-off that she requested.

Her wishes were:

1. Red and white roses only
2. She wanted to be cremated (highly unusual for a Catholic to be cremated most of them believe in burial)
3. Having a Party atmosphere, no crying allowed really only tears of joy, laughter, music, food, more food and cakes.

All this happened as we all pulled it together. It was great to see my best friend Janice. She came by every day. I did not see Tersia as her mum was really unwell, but she came to the funeral service at the church and gave me a great Big Hug.

Janice came by one day and we went to see a friend of hers who lived near us, just down the road and I went with to get out of the house as it was getting really busy.

Her friend was married to a friend of mine from Primary school. This friend mentioned in a joke how I used to wet myself in class.

I was numb and did not say anything at the time (that's the thing with being abused, at times you think you deserve it even though you know better deep down. I did feel the need to stand up for myself, but I was not capable. I will gladly do it for someone else.)

I am still figuring that one out, I am a" work" in walking, thinking and writing progress.

This was a healing time back home in South Africa for me those two weeks with friends and family. Unfortunately, we had to leave on the Sunday when they were burying her ashes with her dad and mum's (my grandfather (Oupa Ben's) and grandmother's (Ouma Betty's),because my husband insisted we leave on the Sunday to be back in Edinburgh on the Monday morning.

I was yearning to stay . . . . My best friend was getting married on New Year's Eve in January 2000. A millennium wedding and I was yearning to be a part of it as she was my maid of honour.

I had to get back though as some friends of mine was coming to spend the millennium in Edinburgh (Nolan and Auntie Cynthie) was visiting so I guess I had to be there and show them around the beautiful and picturesque Edinburgh with its castle in the middle of the town centre. I felt torn.

The guests arrived and I was busy tending to them yet longing for time to grieve mum's death and missing her terribly. I did not speak to anyone about my feelings and I was wanting to be comforted and re-assured. My husband was not offering anything remotely supportive, but my mum-in-law was more attentive and offered a listening ear when I felt like talking, but on the other hand I did not talk too much as I knew she did not have a great relationship with her daughter and I did not want her to feel that she could be my replacement mum. I loved my Mother and I got to understand her a bit more through our adult conversations, actually I was on the phone to her several times within the week before she died and we got closer during my time in the UK.

Becoming a Mother (October 2000)

....

My husband and I decided to start trying for a baby as my dad was getting on in age and I felt that it would be a loss if he did not get to see any of his grandchildren from my line. I stopped taking the contraceptive pills in December. I must have fell pregnant right away because I did not have any period for December or a strange one as it was a "stop-start-spot" one. January came and no period, yay. Pregnancy checks went fine, though I had Rhesus Negative Blood and my husband's was D-positive. Every week I had to have bloods taken at each visit in order to monitor the pregnancy. All went well and on October the 3rd we had a beautiful baby girl and we named her Sophia (pronounced So-fire) a modification of my mum's name who was called Sophy.

His mum was very helpful during the pregnancy, so much so that my opinion did not seem to carry any weight. I kept quiet and allowed this to continue until one day I started questioning her. By then I had become really depressed and did not admit to anyone I was feeling like this. I wanted to breastfeed, but only did this for two weeks as other significant people around me thought that bottle milk was best totally against what we believe in South Africa.

I went back to work early as a result of wanting to be able to go back to South Africa in the summer and if I stayed at home I would not have been able to save up for the ticket costs.

My mother-in-law looked after Sophia, my husband thought it best if she looked after the little one and asked her to give up her day-job in order to do this.

I was torn at the time and could not voice my opinion as I was already seeing problems with the little things she did, which I did not understand as it was the Scottish way of doing things and inside I was screaming out to my mum and missing the way South African coloured interacted with babies, but kept quiet.

By the summer I was really torn between asking for a change or saying nothing. I decided to do a job-share with another teacher at another Primary school in the Borders as the school I was at did not qualify for a job-share.

This worked out a bit better and the arrangements were that my mother-in-law would stay over some nights in order to save her trekking up to Edinburgh from The Borders where we stayed.

She was staying over two nights out of three which meant my daughter and I were not bonding as her nana was always around and she looked to her for comfort. I never felt that I could relax in the house and do what I wanted with Sophia. One night, I have had enough and I asked my mother-in-law to leave that night and she then only came down and drove back up to Edinburgh every night. Sometimes she would take Sophia up to Edinburgh and my husband would go and collect her as he had basketball coaching up some weeknights. Maybe not the best way of doing it and I could have been a bit more tactful, I I was really angry inside and it all boiled over at that point like a slow simmering pot of oats and then it all came gushing out.

We spent most of the weekends up in Edinburgh too because of my husband's coaching commitments and games were played Fridays, Saturdays and Sundays we would go and watch basketball games. I missed seeing my friends and started going up to Edinburgh less. The last incident that really stands out was when I returned from school and I found "custard creams" and "hula hoops" in my cupboards and my mother-in-law explained that it was Sophia's favourite treats. I saw red . . . and felt like someone else is invading my life as the kitchen is my sanctuary and I would not dare go and put foodstuff in someone else's kitchen without checking first.

I told my husband that I was looking for a childminder nearby the school and that at the beginning of the new term the childminder would look after Sophia and that I was tired of being undermined and my wishes not being respected. He had a choice either I would inform his mum or he would.

(I know it was quite strong) My husband said he would do it. Relationships were strained for a while between my husband, his mum and I, but we slotted into our normal patterns after a long period of unease.

She would still try on occasion to be overly helpful, but I was determined to find my own style of parenting.

I specifically knew that both my husband and his mum loved things to be overly neat and tidy so I would leave the kids things lying around and made the home a home.

This used to drive my husband mad and he would always comment on the state of the place when his mum stopped by, but at that point I could not care less. I also noticed how dependent my husband was on his mother and he consulted her on everything and disregarded my opinions or thoughts so I faded away in the background.

The divide grew between my husband and I. He then wanted a second child and I knew then that I did not want a second child into a loveless marriage. I missed taking one of my pills when I was sick and fell pregnant and I was too late to take the morning after pill. (I know not being a good Christian, but I did not want to fall into the same rut)

Sophia on the other hand was diagnosed with Asthma at the age of 8 months and I was already feeling the strain of her needs and was missing having a regular sleep pattern. (I know that does not register once you have children so what am I saying?)

Depression (September 2003-present)

....

At this time I was back to receiving counselling in the Scottish Borders with a lovely lady who worked with the Person-Centred Approach. I worked on my inability to make decisions for myself and my powerlessness and inability to challenge anybody instead of just going along with the flow.

I did not look forward to pregnancy second time round. (Well third time because I did carry Daniel for 21 weeks)

I was also back for more personal therapy to deal with my issues around self-esteem and assertiveness and a lack of self-confidence.

Being a teacher helped me to get out there in front of the children who accept you as you are and do not look at all the flaws I carried inside of me and criticise myself about daily.

I carried and delivered Lemoni on the 4th of January 2003 and it was such a different pregnancy, firstly because I breastfed her up to 6 months, she was crying for most of the first six months of her life and she was a sociable and loving little smiley bundle of joy despite her crying and she adored me.

We slid into backwards mode as a couple because of the lack of sleep and me breastfeeding her so long, I recognised the signs for Postnatal Depression and got help in time and also used that time to receive Art

Therapy where I met a group of amazing women going through exactly what I was experiencing and I did not feel mad anymore as I used to think.

I met two women who I am still friends with one is Japanese lady and the other a Scottish lady.

The cracks were beginning to widen in my marriage and I felt I had to get out.

I left my husband in the April of 2004 for a while and went to temporary accommodation and I really struggled because I did not know anyone and I also did not have much in the means of cash. I told my husband where I was, and he came over (big Mistake on my part) was lovely and it felt so great and I went back. We tried again, but it did not work out. I requested him to work on his issues as I was yet again in therapy working on my issues around standing up for myself and making decisions for myself. I was so scared to make mistakes and make the wrong decisions (dad's words kept coming back: "You are no good, You will never amount to much, "you were nothing but a prostitute for taking money from the abuser")

I wanted him desperately to work on his stuff because I felt I had to give him a last chance even though I knew it was not looking good. He wanted us to go into relationship counselling, but I told him he needed to work on his stuff first.

We went to relationship counselling even though he did not work on his stuff as requested and agreed, but when we got there he wanted us to see a counsellor from a different cultural background as he felt a white counsellor would not understand my issues. I thought this was thoughtful, but looking back it was another ploy of delaying tactics as he was not really interested in seeing anybody in the first place.

I went to this place called Saheliya and saw a lady there who then told me that she could get me a counsellor for myself at the first instance and then I could decide whether I wanted to continue to start the relationship sessions with my husband. Nobody had ever asked me to do that and

I felt; "oh S__t" I can't do this. Making a decision on my own felt alien as I was so used to doing what other people wanted for me even if I disagreed (did not feel I had the energy to challenge, let alone decide)

But I went back to see her as she told me that I did not need to stay with my husband because of my passport stamp. You see one of the things that kept me staying was that my husband used to say that the children were British and I would never be able to take them away as I would be kicked out of the country. I was so scared that I would never be able to see my kids that I stayed as I thought I would be financially dependent on their father. She said that my stamp says it is okay for me to study, work and be legal in this country. I thanked that lady and owe her a lot for opening my eyes. That is another thing when you are in a non-violent but emotionally abusive relationship, you think that you cannot think and you believe everything you are told because you forget that your own opinion counts and always will. I call it "Doormat syndrome"—you function according to someone else's will, wants and needs and yours become flattened as you are being trampled on literally and you cannot see it for a long time as you are so programmed to do as the other party wants that your wants and needs do not register in your brain or mind at all until you are out of that situation. (It may take longer for some or some might never see it)

I received another set of counselling from a person-centred counsellor who was of Japanese origin. Her gentle, non-judgmental manner and calm ways of exploring and helping me make sense of what was going on in the marriage at the time, enabled me to sort out my feelings and needs for myself and the girls. This time I was tired, drained, yet determined to work on that decision I have been sitting with for a long time. To get out and to stay out for my own wellbeing and for the children's wellbeing. I kept thinking what kind of patterns am I teaching my children" that it is okay to be spoken to like you do not matter?"; "That it is okay to be treated like someone with no value?"; "That if you have been sexually abused you have to put up with more abuse?"; "That if your father never loved you, that any kind of love even critical and selfish love would be sufficient?".

I felt that I had better to teach these girls and that they deserve better: respect, love, nurturing, support and most of all to be heard and understood even if people would not always agree with them.

Restoration (September 2004- November 2010)

....

I continued to receive Counselling alongside a set of Complimentary Therapies (Aromatherapy massage) and started to feel like a woman again.

I started a Woman Onto Work Course in September 2004 and started to put my career back on track and to continue the process of restoration I started at Saheliya in April 2004. At the Women Onto Work Course, I started to work on my CV, future plans, but could not decide on a placement (my ghosts of poor decision-making and lack of self-worth was still around). I could not make a decision and then I realised I have been stuck so long in my abuse, abusive childhood, lack of love from my father and mother, poor relationships with men and my poor relationship with myself that I could not think of what I needed, valued and deserved for myself.

I found a placement in a Family Centre in Musselburgh in East Lothian and thoroughly enjoyed it that I knew my dream of becoming a Social Worker or Counsellor was what I wanted to pursue. Of course my husband encouraged me at the beginning and after that he would be so negative and critical about it that I stopped sharing my dreams in case it acquired doormat syndrome too.

Later on I realised that the decision I have been sitting on for the past 4 years is going to happen and the second-last day of the course I broke down because I realised after doing an exercise of the most stressful situations, that I had most of them happen within a year . . . 1. moved country; 2. moved house; 3. I gave birth the year before; 4. I had postnatal depression; 5. I Lost a parent; 6. Changed career; 7. I had little support around me.

I was still petrified about making this decision and where would I start to explain to my dad mostly as he thought the world of my husband. I knew my sister and my friends would understand as I have been unhappy for a long time now. All the parents at nursery, all the basketball people, all the family and family friends . . . what do you say? where do you start?

I had so many what ifs in my mind? What happens if I meet someone from Basketball? Do I still go to Basketball? Do I stop going altogether because I was so saturated with it all??What do I say and most of all what do I do?

I decided on Christmas day after watching the interaction between my then husband, his mum and dad and my children. It was such struggle to get money for the shopping and the other necessities for the whole day that I felt so embarrassed to be asking in front of my in-laws that I felt this would be the last time I will be putting my kids and I through this torture.

Of course there was no problem with getting the alcohol . . . .

My husband regularly put his mum down and was really rude with her, I had to walk away and go and count to 100 a few times and also wondered at the same time "why would someone allow their child to speak to them in that manner?"

My New Year's gift to myself would be peace away from this destructive relationship which I also had a part in as I allowed all this to happen because of my poor communication skills. I wanted to acknowledge that I had a part to play in allowing the relationship to get to this stage.

I needed a change and I wanted it this year and that was the difference as I made that decision and not somebody else. I usually let someone else decide because I was too scared to make a mistake and then I would have someone to blame.

I did not want to blame people anymore and I made a decision to take responsibility for my own actions and decisions. I allowed myself to become subservient, docile and compliant in order not to go through the arguments in front of the kids, I had to focus on the ultimate goal of getting out of the relationship and not causing more damage for the children as I wanted so much more for them than what I had with their father. I was receiving support from a women's organisation called SHAKTI women's aid and they assisted me with all the practical and emotional advice since in April 2004. I put a plan together with the support worker as I just did not want to up sticks and go so I planned it for the December period when I knew my husband would be away and I made that all important phone call on the 27th of December to my Support worker and got all our stuff together while my husband was away taking his mum down south to his sister's.

I knew it was cowardly and I also knew that if I waited he would have persuaded me to stay and we could work things out like the last time . . . and last time only lasted for two weeks and then it went back to how things were before then. This is not what I wanted for myself and my children as I felt then that I would be teaching them that it is okay to be treated like someone with no independent thought for themselves and no respect between husband and wife; male and female or any relationship where one person has more power over the other. I believe in having equal power and a power-sharing relationship, yes at times one of you preferably the male will override a decision even though both of you offered your viewpoints and in some instances it would work the other way too where the other partner would override a decision made together as circumstances may have changed since the decision was last made.

I left on the 29th of December 2004 with £2 in my wallet, three sports bags with our clothes for a week and my files with all the personal information and certificates I have acquired in South Africa and the United Kingdom.

I moved back to Edinburgh because all the support was here from the Women's Aid and I guess a sense of familiarity. It was culturally more diverse (for the kids and myself) we were living in a predominantly white village with only a few people from different cultural backgrounds, in East Lothian and I wanted the girls to have a bit more exposure to different people.

Those first weeks were tough. I decided not to speak to my husband when he phoned to speak to the girls within those first two weeks as I knew I would go back if I heard him beg and say all the usual things he said to get me back.

The friends that were around at the time were fantastic. I had two close friends in the Borders (my friend Leonie from New Zealand who lived in the Borders and we had our children in the same year met whilst and they would take it in turns to phone me, come up and see us and take me out to get some bits and pieces as being on benefits was quite restrictive financially.

At night times though it was awful as I could not get to sleep and the little one (Lemoni) was a restless sleeper and would not settle, she would sleep for a few hours and then wake up constantly. Later on the only way she would sleep was if I was next to her and that was tiring as it meant I would not get a decent night's sleep with her tossing and turning and stroking me all the time (she did this thing where she would stroke my breast and then later on after it became embarrassing and also I felt it was becoming a dependency habit) I started to divert her hand up to my neck and she could stroke that part, I reckoned that it had the same texture as my breast and she could then be weaned off gradually. Maybe she found comfort after missing being breastfed, I do not know, she still does it (she calls it nee nees).

We stayed in temporary accommodation for a month and a half and was offered a brand new flat with Port Of Leith Housing Association near The Shore. This was a lovely flat and was also near the school so quite handy really. I was still receiving support from Shakti Women's Aid with regards to legal advice, benefits, debts, training opportunities and a great deal of support through the Children's workers. There were outings, children's activities on Fridays and family outings in Spring and Summer, it was amazing and very well geared to give the women a vision to look ahead and also that we can still function as families, a bit different, but we could still go and engage with the wider community with our children and not narrow or limit our sights because we do not have a male figure in our lives any more.

The girls still had contact with their dad and I felt that that was important and also not to bad mouth their dad in front of them, sometimes it did slip out at the beginning stages, but I always felt their hurt, my shame and disappointment with myself for letting myself down.

Deep down I am a really nice person, but I have toughened myself up in order to protect myself because I DID NOT WANT TO BE TAKEN ADVANTAGE OF, BUT ALONG THE WAY I LOST THE ABILITY TO REASON AND RECOGNISE WHEN IT WENT TOO FAR AND WAS NOT REALLY NECESSARY AND SOME OF MY RESPONSES WERE WAY TOO WEIRD TO UNDERSTAND. I WAS VERY DEFENSIVE AND TOOK ME A LONG TIME TO WORK ON THE REASONS I TOLD MYSELF TO BE THAT WAY IN ORDER TO JUSTIFY MY BEHAVIOUR AND RESPONSES. I CAN STILL BE DESCRIBED AS BLUNT, TOO DIRECT AND CURT AT TIMES, BUT I WOULD LIKE TO THINK THAT I AM BECOMING MUCH SOFTER AND MORE LIKE A HUGGABLE MARSHMALLOW.

As they say in my friendship circles, I am under construction.

Legal proceedings were started, but my solicitor advised me to wait for a year as it will speed the process up and I could consider if this is what I really wanted and then after the Marriage has broken down and we tried all options available to us I can then proceed with formal paperwork.

It was a lovely lady from Balfour and Manson a highly established legal firm in Edinburgh and I was pleased with the way things were being dealt with.

During that time contact arrangements were put in place in order that the girls would still see their dad.

The girls saw their dad on a Tuesday and every other Thursday through to Sunday evenings when they would be returned at 6pm and we shared most holidays. I still did not trust their dad to get them ready for school and Lemoni was starting Nursery soon so I wanted to make sure they looked presentable. That is the South African in me as a lot of value is placed on appearance and how you present yourself and your children. Of course I now know that is a very stereotypical outlook and allow the children to choose how they present themselves with a little bit of guidance. I also inform them that just because someone is not all coordinated, not dressed like everyone else and looks the same, it does not make them a bad person and different and creative is a good thing.

We were put together by my mother to be all nice and coordinated as the comments will go back to. "did you see what miss Canary's daughter was wearing yesterday, what a disgrace . . . half cut denim shorts with holes in them, scruffy trainers (Tekkies) and the rest . . . . (a very Coloured approach). (I mean no disrespect to people of colour, but this is the term I have associated myself with and grew up with in My hometown of Port Elizabeth in South Africa), I feel if I start saying mixed race it puts me in another state of identity crisis and the Apartheid years have messed a lot with my mind already regarding race, value, acceptance and levels of attainment and expectancy).

Coloured stayed in my mind as I am a bit of my Gran's Tamal Indian, My grandpa's very dark coloured roots, my dad's white heritage (mixed) and my mum's mixed heritage). We are all inter-mixed the way I see it. As my daughters and I say (Merry Mix). (Again I must emphasize that we mean no disrespect to any race, culture or country).

I could not get beyond this point for a long time as I was starting to get flashbacks and memories as if they were happening in the here and now. I had to take good care of myself and go for long walks to keep my head in a healthy space as it is so easy to go back in the hole and not want to come out. I used to comfort eat, now see it as a form of self harm as I loathe my body and the only way I could feel better would be to overeat anything (chocolates (dark chocolate not really my favourite I prefer milk chocolate, biscuits—a packet of custard creams, maybe a few digestives or shortbread, bread—white toast is the best or fresh tiger bread with lots of butter and fish paste (Peck's Anchovette from South Africa, food—leftover or freshly cooked/anything I could find really as I did not really register what was going in just that at those moments I could not stop to fill this hole and I did not have the natural responses to know when to stop as it was overridden by the emotional pain I felt at the time.

Then I have to struggle with the feelings of guilt after I have been binging and that is then far worse because of all the good work I would do through exercise, keeping fit for about three months and looking and feeling a little better about myself and my body. Then feeling dirty, cheap and sexy and not being able to deal with the admiring glances from men and women because of my inner voices of shame, guilt, feelings of unworthiness and ugliness (because I was never told I am beautiful or valuable from my parents).

In 2007 I enrolled in a part-time counselling diploma in person-centred counselling at the University of Strathclyde upon completion of a Counselling certificate with support from the manager of the Mental health organisation in Edinburgh and with encouragement from my then colleagues. The interviews were being held in February of 2008 and would start in September 2008.I was accepted, s__t, I thought as I was not expecting to get in. I got lost on the day and was 5 minutes late because I was too embarrassed to ask anybody and only asked someone from the library that looked reasonably friendly, and was already nervous because it was such a big, impressive building, never thought I would go to university anywhere (let alone in the United Kingdom). This was a course based on experiential learning through being yourself and learning as yourself. At first I thought "no I cannot do this." As usual I was placing all these obstacles in my own path of self-destruction by thinking negative thoughts.

I was the only person of colour and I do have a thing about large numbers and feeling unsafe, but I told myself that I would challenge myself and take on small risks related to changing how I think, feel and operate as most of my beliefs still stemmed from an upbringing in South Africa within the context of a coloured neighbourhood. I did not strive for much and was not hoping to achieve much after being a primary teacher, yet I longed within to be somebody amazing and wonderful, but never thought to say this out loud as I thought people would just burst out laughing at me.

I worked with a counsellor at a place called Link-Up women's support centre in Restalrig Edinburgh on feelings of self worth and acceptance as I was beginning to question my relationships and why I could not seem to make it work beyond the 4 month mark and why was this happening and what was really going on within me. At the time I was also experiencing quite a few complications with regard to my work relationships and doubted my abilities to perform at work and was experiencing high stress levels at the workplace.

This was really confusing to me as my life was supposed to be back on track now: in my head it was all sorted; 1. Sexual abuse done; 2. Father dead all memories and feelings of low self-worth done; 3. Attitudes and feelings of being good enough done and dealt with; 4. girls and I getting things back on track in order to provide continuity as things were happening at their father's I was not happy with; 5. Loving boyfriend/ partner who loves me for who I am; 6. life was looking a hell of a lot better than a year ago. I operated on a tick list system and hoped that once it received a tick in my mind, that was it done and ready to be boxed away.

Somehow it still felt like I was looking back all the time and I wanted to know what was going on inside me. I Was going into a downward spiral again and even though everything seemed to be working well in my favour (girls and I are getting along better, Banji loved me even though I a mess at times, my career is getting on track, my friendships are solid). I was still overeating at night, where it used to be bread and junk food now I SEEM TO SUBSTITUTE IT WITH HEALTHY FOOD (RICE CRACKERS, BERRIES, DARK CHOCOLATE, SESAME SNAPS, ALMONDS, DRIED FRUIT AND THE LIST GOES ON). I would go to the gym, work out for an hour, feel great, then at night when I look at myself and the kids have gone to bed I start eating. I never really felt that I am an attractive, sexy woman and all attention always related to sex and the sexual abuse. The attention, even compliments from women put me in an awkward place and I never knew how to react as it put me under the invisible spotlight. Dad never gave me compliments either and I never knew what it was to accept compliments and not feel that you have to do anything in return to earn the compliment because I felt worthless and of no value.

I can very easily give compliments in order to make someone feel good and genuinely feel good about giving the compliment, still I felt uneasy to receive it. I am getting better at accepting the compliment without being expected to do any favour in return.

My hair is a subject of joy, pride and also shame, disgust and self-loathing.

When dad told me that I looked like a prostitute at the age of 15, it stuck. It affected how I styled my hair, sometimes I left my hair naturally curly and frizzy to rebel against him and also to get a reaction from him and my mum. Later on I started to self-harm by cutting it short, straightening it, dying it black or dark brown, relaxing it and then also shaving it off. I thought if I look like a boy then men won't notice me then I would not have to worry about how I looked. I gained a lot of weight and I thought that if I cover up the sexual curviness of my feminine shape then I would not have to deal with the attention and care that comes with being a woman and then also it saved me from having to look at how I am mistreating my body.

At times I still wish to be skinny and not have big breasts (32 K) highly disproportionate because my frame is actually small. In my mind it meant that I could then pretend to be androgynous and not draw attention to myself as I do not like the attention. I hated my hourglass figure because it is so feminine and womanly even if I try to gain weight and hide it or lose the weight to be healthy. I love being healthy and feeling good, but then I have to admit that I am attractive and a beautiful human being created by God. The shift came when I had to look at my whole issues of self-control, self-acceptance and love for myself. I mean how do you explain to yourself that God loves you even though I have been sexually abused, messed-up, unhappy, unworthy and fat.

When I shifted the thinking processes of acceptance by God my creator and Father, I had to look at the reasons behind my thinking and how it started How can I be a daughter to God when my own dad never made me feel like the little princess I so often see dads do to their daughters. That look of love and admiration from the dads when they interact with their daughters, is a wonderful thing to observe and admire. I worked through it with my counsellor at Link-Up I had to learn accept that my frame is curvy and I am a beautiful, striking woman (I still cringe when I say that and think about it) but it is getting better.

Having found God as a true father and comforter I am a work in progress.

A friend of mine who I was working with me in the voluntary sector at the time in 2007, invited me to her church and I was thinking up a new excuse each time when she asked, but she never gave up, so I went in February 2007 to a service at Destiny Church in Leith. Amy was always very good at checking out my opinion about favourite women's topics and I found her confident, open and assertive manner quite refreshing with her lovely polished English accent. She was really interested in listening to the women's voices and made the time and effort to have their views put across. We had some interesting chats at work during our lunch and coffee breaks. Later on we extended the coffee breaks out with the office and we still meet up regularly for Soya Lattes and Soya hot chocolates in lovely, quirky coffee shops in Edinburgh. You see, I always thought that a certain kind of person would be allowed into these coffee shops because of my lack of and low self-esteem and no confidence. (Amy walked in with her confident stride, head held high and never commented on my unease and my constant looking around and comparing myself with the rest of the coffee, tea and hot chocolate consumers.) Secretly, I wished I could be like that and I am now like that thanks to Amy.

I quite liked it and thought okay I will go back as it was a little bit, okay a lot different from the Catholic church I grew up in South Africa. I went back and decided to commit in April 2007. I attended Amy's wedding service in July 2008 and saw a few familiar faces from Destiny at her wedding. Amy attended my baptism in Destiny Church on September 13th 2009 and we still share a friendship that is growing all the time.

The girls and I still bump into Amy and her husband at Destiny services. She continues to be patient with my insecurities, recently she pulled me up on selling myself short in my counselling and workshop flyer and she told me that I am too humble and shy and that I should sell myself more as I she thinks that I am an amazing woman. (I am under construction)

Marie Biscuit

I met Caryn when she was studying at The University of Edinburgh at the centre for African Studies (Food marketing) and completed and RECEIVED HER doctorate last year November. (she is now Doctor Caryn Abrahams). I met her in church one Sunday and she could pick up on my South African accent. I was not that keen to meet up with South Africans in case they knew anybody from back home and my stuff would be spread around in South Africa and I was very guarded, but I sensed that she might be different so I accepted when she invited me for a coffee.

South Africa is a small place where people like to gossip especially about people's downfalls and I wanted to spare my family the hassle. She turned out to be a strong force in my discovery of God, although she is young, she understood me and she has a unswerving belief in God. She was pivotal in making me commit to the Baptism and taking the next step to becoming a Born again Christian. Her talk about being a Marie biscuit (Rich Tea biscuit) in stead of a chocolate covered fancy biscuit still comes to mind when I was questioning her about the gooey, goose bumpy feelings I used to feel at the beginning of my journey to Christianity and she quickly pointed out that actually a plain prayer is just as effective as the elaborate prayers and we all pray to the same God, but sometimes we get too caught up in the fancy side trimmings that we forget the basic, simple origins and that can lead us astray when we lose our focus. She is my Marie biscuit (Rich Tea) reminder of staying grounded and keeping it simple and real and not trying too hard to be someone else because I think my contribution is not valuable.

My Faith now has also lead me to become a full member of Destiny church and now serving on the staff team to help out as a volunteer counsellor.

This has been a slow and very humbling experience being able to support people in their own personal journeys to overcome personal struggles and also have a safe space to talk about things in confidence as the church can sometimes be an unsafe place to be if you think everyone knows your 'stuff'.

It is now then that I realise I have discovered my Faith but not in a conventional way and I am still searching, but now I am on track to a closer and more real relationship with God.

This has also given me an opportunity to start dipping into the Women's workshops and seminars I would love to run for women and their relationships with themselves and God.

I am now beginning to start looking into developing the counselling service and opening up to all people from all backgrounds religious and no belief system at all and also a service for the youth as I believe in preventative work that would ultimately give young people safe spaces to talk about all their feelings and experiences and to facilitate them in their own understanding of themselves.

Beautiful Potter (Scotland)

Coffee and hugs come to mind when it honk of Yvette. We met about 6 years ago at multicultural group called the Rainbow group. I used to look at the information when I first started coming to Edinburgh in 1998 and always felt that I would like to go but because I did not have a family I felt I could not go.

This place was a great place to go to especially on Sunday afternoons when I did not know what else or who else to go to with the girls as I have not made any friends due to my lack of trust and not wanting anybody to know my business and ask lots of questions.

I saw this lady there who could be a coloured from the Northern suburbs in South Africa and warmed to her. She was beautiful, confident, same complexion as myself and had a mixed race son. She was smiley, very intelligent and I thought to myself "I would like to become her friend", but somehow the little voice came back to tell me "she won't want to be around me ". I stalled and thought I will wait till the next meeting in two weeks time and see if I can muster up the courage to ask her to meet for a coffee. I asked her the next time as we decided it was a nice enough day to take the children to the park afterwards. It turned out that she knew my friend Bertha who left the August before. We met up for coffee a few weeks after that and hit it off really apart from the fact that she was a healthy vegetarian (no-meat eating kind) the kind I always dreamt of but never quite got it together because South Africans are brought up with meat and meat and meat. I tried to be vegetarian once and only ate fish, bad idea my mum told me I would need to take vitamin supplements as I already had low blood counts.

I was really weak and was getting sick of boiled vegetables, fruit salad toast and rice. AFTER WATCHING Yvette cook vegetarian food I am convinced it is an alternative and I ACTUALLY ENJOY HER FOOD! AND SHE CAN BAKE CAKES! I have not been baking cakes and biscuits as I was still using cups and spoon measurements and trying to "guesstimate" the ingredient so it always came out funny, so I gave up, but Yvette told me to get a scale that has both pounds and ounces and kilograms and milligrams on it and she showed me a couple of easy recipes to start me off. Now I can bake with my girls, Yay!

She is a very disciplined person and always watches what she puts in her mouth very carefully where I just eat after the taste and think about the effects later on . . . I mean way later . . . . (You know what I mean)

With the result that I am always wondering what to wear and if it will still fit me whereas Yvette can just go to het cupboard and pick what she needs to wear and it will fit.

I attempt to go to the gym twice a week, Yvette makes sure she goes three to four times a week. It felt that I knew Yvette for a long time and I invited her for a coffee somewhere in Leith at Embo's. I always wanted to go there, but I did not feel I had the confidence to go in alone. I felt Yvette would be right at home in such a kind of funky, Arty Farty Coffee shop and she did. I was not wrong.

We talked about lots of different topics and I was at the time pursued by a distinguished gentleman and I felt I could talk to her about him. He was however with somebody else and I felt that she did not judge me as I struggled to make up my mind about whether to accept his advances or not.

She could be a great counsellor if she was interested, but I do not think she is.

We are still friends and she is pivotal in keeping me from doubting myself when I am doing great and I suddenly feel . . . 'woaw' things are getting too good too fast.

Her utter objective honesty has kept me from making reactive decisions in the heat of the moment and to re-think instead to make responsible decisions.

We have known each other for over 6 years, but it feels like a lifetime.

And you know what, she always encourages me and never makes me feel like the fat girlfriend. She comments on what I wear and compliments my natural curvy shape. A true friend is what she is.

When I was told that for my graduation I am only allowed two guests but could have a spare ticket I thought of Yvette and Banji and one other friend, but this was so difficult as there were so many friends who supported me during my two years at University. I chose Theresa as both her and Frank has been there listening to my woes on Wednesday evenings, Friday evenings and over Saturday or Sunday dinners when they would invite me round when the girls were away at their dad's.

She does not like driving on the motorway, but because I asked her to attend my graduation (4th November 2010, she did it (even though it was raining and my directions were c___p).

Gadget Girl

Kuwait—South Africa

My friends have become my family and I have a few significant friends, Tersia Assumption who I met at Teacher Training College and I had a connection with. I thought she was a Bad A__s chick and I wanted to be like her. She is confident, smart and she takes no S__t from nobody and the thing that stands out for me is her ability to stand up to my mother and not allow my mum to stop our friendship. Mum had a habit of choosing my friends and did not allow me to go anywhere near the once she thought was not good for me without even giving them a chance. This was very frustrating while I was attending teacher's college. She could not come to my house as mum did not approve of our friendship. We met outwith and I lied to get out of the house (18) and I was always welcome at her family home and her sisters' homes. Tersia is now teaching in Kuwait and we still text each other every other day, spend time on SKYPE when the technology plays along, visits every other year or so. She came over in July 2008 and it was great as we spent time together exploring Scotland on day trips and resting mostly as I was on a low budget and could not really spend that much, but it was just great to have a familiar face and speak Afrikaans and hang out.

We have been friends for over 20 years and still going strong even though mum did not approve. I guess I had a sense of my own mind and who I wanted to be friends with.

New Zealand—Scotland

I met Leonie Sole while I was doing Supply Teaching in Edinburgh. She was very friendly, approachable and easy to talk to. We met regularly for coffee, drinks at the weekends and when I was struggling to get a teaching job, she recommended me to her head teacher and I was hired.

I think of Leonie as a vegetarian, strong yet gentle, well educated, well read, open-minded and a strong sense of what's right and wrong and no B___l S__t.

I spent a lot of time with her when we both lived in Edinburgh, but then I moved to the Borders where My then husband and I both secured permanent jobs.

Not long after that we both fell pregnant and then had our first children Leonie had Theo in August of 2000 and I had Sophia in October 2000.

The friendship continued and I guess we struck a connection and we found out we had similar childhood experiences and experiences of Scotland coming in as foreigners from another country of birth, trying to hold on to our family values and yet trying to integrate our children into the Scottish culture and yet trying to teach them some of our own countries inheritance we grew up with.

Leonie was one of the first friends to notice the change in me when things were not that great with my marriage and how I struggled to hide my feelings and struggles.

She supported me to be true so myself and decide for myself and to start making decisions for myself. I look back and realise that I took some of Tersia's guts and Leonie's gumption to finally make a decision to leave the ALREADY SHIPWRECKED MARRIAGE.

Banji—Trinidad /Nigeria—UK

I met Banji on an internet dating website called E-Harmony, being such a stickler for questions and thorough checklists I felt it would be a great place to find someone. I somehow thought, if they are as thorough as the questionnaires, then surely the guys will be thorough (My thoughts at the time . . . somehow it has shifted, thank goodness for that)

He is originally British born (Half Nigerian (dad) and half Trinidadian (mum) and was looking for a Christian woman of below the 40 aged mark as he wanted children . . . . (I know it sounds like a cattle call advert) Mature cow, in good condition, must have . . . strong hips, child bearing age . . . . European . . . you know what I mean . . .

I was really just goofing around before University started really and was not that serious as I always went for the far away guys in the States (USA—United States of America), the Caribbean—all my sisters who had brothers were all happy with their Caribbean men so I reckoned I want one of them and that is that!! I did not want anybody from the African continent as I had a few interesting experiences which left me a bit weary. (I know it sounds judgmental, but if you meet me, you will know that I am not judgemental in the least, I used to be and I blame my South African messed up Apartheid brainwashing and ignorance inherited from my dad, but I thank God for my mother who was a forward thinking open-minded individual when it came to meeting and socialising with people)

After the questions and security measures in place we went to open communication. Now I must admit the time difference did throw me for a bit, but then I realised they were behind times so it worked out to my advantage.

We started open communication for a while after September and continued, but then I started Uni (university) and I also did not really have my heart set on finding a bloke on a computer. (come on how was I to know the dude was not just pretending to be someone he was not or he looked nothing like his picture (half the people seemed to post pictures that were take n 10 years earlier and did not reflect at all what they resemble in real life!).I was a terrible communicator really, but the guy was determined and nudged me a couple of times.

Eventually after November I sent him a message along these lines: "Hi there, I am sorry I have not been communicating for a while, but if you have not given up on me, here is my email. I look forward to your reply, if you have found someone then the best of luck. Take care Jazz (Jacintha)"

I left it and then in January I got something from him and we chatted via facebook at first and then moved on to Skype (another foreign concept!!) Technology is not one of my strengths . . . . I had two MP3 players (one Theresa gave me and the other one Tersia gave me). I only use them for few weeks then they find their way to the bottom of my basket where I put all my notes and special cards and stuff . . . do you get me??

Skype was a challenge to download, but I got some help from Rania a lovely Egyptian lady who was studying at Edinburgh University doing her PhD and who was at home with technology as she had to do everything on her computer (notes, statistics, interviews and a, lot more) who I met through Caryn and she talked me through the instructions. I persisted I felt something different about Banji and he was really good at keeping in touch, I would receive a morning call, evening and weekends were great as it was 5 hours behind . . . so lunchtime here would be morning for him. We communicated from January 02 2010 and then I asked him in March if he would like to come over as it would have been too long to wait till August when he would be relocating for good to London. Secretly I felt that if he said "No" then he was not really that interested, but if he said

"Yes" then he must be into me. I was really into him, but I did not tell him that of course.

He came over in April 2010 for a week and a bit and we really struck up some kind of connection. I took him around to meet some of my friends because in my head we were already committed and . . . and a very important part of the girls and my life. The introductions to my friends were really an extension of accepting him into my life and to illustrate how important he was to me. This did not work out so well in the end as Banji is extremely private and he does not specifically choose to socialise in small or large group settings.

Looking back I should have been a bit more sensitive to his needs and noises he made regarding meeting people and socialising as a whole. Not a proud moment, I could not see anything wrong at the time and chose not to apologise, but later on after a lot of discussions over Skype and chats when he came over in November 2010 I apologised and we negotiated that I should respect his wishes when he declines a social engagement. I still find it difficult to accept as I am such a social, hospitable and generous spirit.

I am hoping that Banji will learn to be comfortable around the people that I bring into my church community, friends and the strays which I love to nurture and love.

We are still in the first stages of our relationship as we are getting to know each other's intricacies and quirks (and there are a lot on my side . . . and he has a few too . . . .) but it feels comfortable and I will focus on that for now. We are taking things slow and we will see where God leads us from here

My love for Banji is tender yet strong as the thought of him just moves me to such tender tears and my heart wells up when I think of him.

On the other side of that tenderness is the frustration and somehow the day to day faith and endurance that keeps people together for a length of time when the human side of me is not in line with my Christlike self that focuses on being patient, loving, compassionate and forgiving.

The girls

I would fight anybody who harms my children.

I would also forgive them if they do the unthinkable, because I am somebody transformed and changed within.

Two really opposing thoughts and I am left with trusting in God to steer me in the right direction as I know my children are not mine to possess, but they will become their own person.

My love for the girls are filled with sunshine, steadfast endurance and a strong pain threshold as I can be moved to tears when I just look at them. Even though I have a sergeant Major approach with them (they can see right through it though) I do not know who am I kidding, I guess it keeps me centred and when I have to go to hospitals and deal with pain (school, friends, the community and life) I can be strong for them.

Love

Firstly I love God, myself, Banji, my children (god daughter), my family (in my own way), my nieces, my friends, my fellow colleagues (the special ones) and I love children as I have an affinity for all children.

I have changed my attitude to love quite significantly over the past four years as I had to learn how to love myself and treat myself nicely, kindly, gently, lovingly and I had to learn this in order for me to understand and accept myself.

It has been a struggle, I still find receiving compliments hard, but I accept them now whereas before I would not even respond at all.

Love is important to me as it has taught me to be gentle with myself and accept all the parts of me (the 9 year old, the confident woman, the strong mother, the insecure mother, the good friend, the assertive friend, the loving girlfriend, the supportive girlfriend, the angry 9 year old, the angry woman re-discovering herself, the angry teenager, the rebellious young adolescent, the lovely bubbly gentle woman, the hurt woman, the survivor, the fighter, the campaigner for young women and the fair and honest woman).

The love has enabled me to be true to myself and go with the spoken rather than the unspoken and also allowed me to take risks in the groups and with individuals as it was very important to stay true to myself at all times and not to become someone I did not recognise anymore.

Love is exciting, hurtful, special, sensitive, tiring, empowering, tender and most of all freeing. I look at love with a rich, open-minded approach and I can bend with the gentle breezes, the strong gusts of wind, the unexpected storms and most of all the little unexpected surprises that it brings and makes my whole being come alive and tingle with ripples of goose bumps all over and inside my body when I think of all the special people that make my world and life that it is.

There is a special piece of love pie for all the special people in my life, God gets the biggest piece, Banji, the girls, my family and friends, children, women and men around the world.

The tapestry is started and it will continue as I evolve in myself, with God, with Banji, with my girls, my friends and sisters, the community and life out there.

I want to thank you, the reader for choosing this book and for reading it. Having survived sexual abuse, it has been a liberating experience to put my experiences in words and to re-start my life as an individual after feeling trapped and restricted by not being allowed to tell my story when my dad told me not to tell anyone and to keep it in the family. This re-inforced t he ideas and thoughts that I was to blame and at fault. A message that lingered with me all this time for the best part of my life and stopped me from forming meaningful relationships as I could never feel totally at ease with myself. I can finally say that I can start my life after being told to put it on hold for 29years. My 39th birthday present to myself is freedom to be a worthy and valued individual who has a lot to offer and a lot to learn in life on my journey.

Once again a heartfelt thank you for reading my story.

A few significant quotes which helped me stay on the path of recovery to better Mental Health

> A Child given the opportunity has the gift of honest, forthright communication. (Anonymous/Unknown)

> A Mother who is respected and accepted with dignity can also be sincerely expressive when she knows that she will not be criticised and blamed. (Anonymous)

> We are all doing our BEST.
> The Best Is All We Can Do.
> Life is going to be All Right.
> Life will be All Right.
>
> (Anonymous/Unknown)

Sexual abuse

This is when a child is used sexually by an adult or young person. Making a child look at pornographic magazines or films is also sexual abuse. Sexual abuse is when a child or young person is pressurised, forced or tricked into taking part in any kind of sexual activity with an adult or young person. This can include kissing, touching the young person's genitals or breasts, intercourse or oral sex.

Who sexually abuses children?

Child sex abusers:
- can come from any professional, racial or religious background, and can be male or female
- are not always adults—children and young people can also behave in a sexually abusive way
- are usually known to the child—they may be a family member or a family friend.

How do they operate?

Abusers may act alone or as part of an organised group. They sometimes prefer children of a particular age, sex, physical type or ethnic background.

After the abuse, they may put the child under great pressure not to tell anyone about it. They often go to great lengths to get close to children and win their trust. For example by:

- choosing employment that brings them into contact with children
- pretending to be children in internet chat rooms run for children and young people.

Child sex abusers are sometimes referred to as "paedophiles" or "sex offenders", especially when they are not family members.
(NSPCC website)

Music that helped me along the way

M People—Search for a Hero
Kirk Franklin—STOMP
Ayiesha Woods—Happy
Chris Tomlin—How Great is our God
Whitney Houston—The Greatest Love of All
Gloria Gaynor—I Will Survive
Israel Houghton—Moving forward
Josh Groban—You Raise Me Up
India Arie—I Am Not My Hair

Afterword

I told this story in order to break the silence that kept me trapped for 29 years as a result of the sexual abuse during my childhood. I could not move on and it has been a long and difficult time. It still is at times, I am not trying to make it sound like everything is now fixed, there are still days that cripple me and it is hard to get out of bed, see meaning in life and forge ahead, but those days are getting less.
The hope and healing is a stronger force in my life and motivates me to encourage and support anybody who needs it.
Sexual abuse is wrong!
It is so damaging, not only when you are a child, but it also limits your quality of life in the later years.
Children are our gifts and reminders to be care free and full of smiles and should be treated with love, care and respect.

In writing this my aim is to work together with young people and women (and men) to look at the gifts God has in store for us and to reach out and bless others as we are meant to be to one another.

Jacintha J. Canary